Basic Science
for
Dental Auxiliaries

Basic Science for Dental Auxiliaries

CLARINDA E. OLSON
Seattle Central Community College

PRENTICE-HALL, INC., Englewood Cliffs, New Jersey 07632

Library of Congress Cataloging in Publication Data

Olson, Clarinda E.
    Basic science for dental auxiliaries.

    Bibliography: p.
    1. Dentistry. 2. Teeth. 3. Anatomy, Human.
4. Human physiology. 5. Dental auxiliary personnel.
I. Title. [DNLM: 1. Dental auxiliaries. 2. Head—
Anatomy and histology. 3. Neck—Anatomy and histology.
4. Tooth—Anatomy and histology. WU101.3 052b]
RK280.047   612'.31'0236176   78-9854
ISBN 0-13-069245-X

Editorial/production supervision: Eleanor Henshaw Hiatt
Cover design: Richard Lo Monaco
Manufacturing buyer: Cathie Lenard

Printed in the United States of America
10 9 8 7 6 5 4 3 2 1

PRENTICE-HALL INTERNATIONAL, INC., *London*
PRENTICE-HALL OF AUSTRALIA PTY. LIMITED, *Sydney*
PRENTICE-HALL OF CANADA, LTD., *Toronto*
PRENTICE-HALL OF INDIA PRIVATE LIMITED, *New Delhi*
PRENTICE-HALL OF JAPAN, INC., *Tokyo*
PRENTICE-HALL OF SOUTHEAST ASIA PTE. LTD., *Singapore*
WHITEHALL BOOKS LIMITED, *Wellington, New Zealand*

This book is dedicated
to my very patient husband, Howard,
who never once complained
during the two years I was married to my typewriter.

Contents

5

MICROORGANISMS AND STERILIZATION 209

Preface

Although I am not a scientist, I am a student of science who is intensely interested in the subject. For many years I have taught the life sciences to dental auxiliary students at Seattle Central Community College. My teaching led to many hours of study, of course, and as the years went by, I began to wonder how much background in the life sciences was needed to ensure optimum performance as a dental auxiliary. The question ultimately led to this simplified book.

One of the problems facing dentistry today is the lack of qualified auxiliaries who can be trained in the shortest possible time. With the advent of "legalized functions," the one- and two-year curricula have been expanded. Therefore, this text attempts to combine and simplify the life sciences that are required in accredited dental auxiliary courses, so that more time can be spent on training auxiliaries to perform the legalized functions.

New words and their definitions appear at the end of each subsection, and many short self-tests allow the readers to check their understanding of the material they have studied.

I hope the readers—whether students or interested browsers—find this simplified text interesting and informative.

Clarinda E. Olson

Acknowledgments

Many of my associates have encouraged me to complete this text and have contributed constructive criticism. To them I am grateful. Without their interest I could not have dedicated two years of my life to this book.

Three persons: Barbara Mercer, R.N.; Aileen Anderson; and Melvin F. Rugg, D.D.S. receive special recognition for the many long hours they spent in making suggestions, and in reading and correcting my manuscript.

C. E. O.

Basic Science
for
Dental Auxiliaries

1

Anatomy and Physiology

THE GENERAL DESIGN OF THE HUMAN BODY

Anatomy and physiology are best understood if the reader is somewhat familiar with the theory of man's beginnings. However, one must remember that as each year passes, new discoveries and new theories will be forthcoming. To someone in a future society, today's theories may be as archaic as those of the distant past. Thus, you should think of this brief review of anatomy and physiology as a beginning—as only a step to a further in-depth study of man.

Many hypotheses have been proposed about the earth's and man's origins. If the calendar of events covering the earth's billions of years were to be condensed into one year, it would appear to have happened something like the following:

January	Earth began in a cloud of cosmic dust.
July	Earliest signs of life occurred.
November	Earth's atmosphere was now such that it could support life, and lower forms of life became abundant.
December	As time went on and conditions on earth warranted, land plants, reptiles, and mammals became abundant, and then, on the last day of December—man appeared.

Eventually it became apparent that much was to be learned about the many millions of individual organisms that inhabited the earth, but it was found impossible to study each organism separately. A system of classification had to be invented. This was a difficult task. The Greek philosopher and biologist Aristotle (384—322 B.C.) was the first, to our knowledge, to discuss separating the various species; and although at that time there were only a few hundred known kinds of animals and plants, Aristotle still was faced with the problem of how to classify them. Should they be classified by species or by common attributes? With the help of a student, Aristotle did succeed, to some extent, in making a general classification according to species.

In time, man, as one of the individual organisms that needed classification, was categorized as belonging to the animal kingdom, the Mammalia class, order of Primates, Hominidae family (resembling man), genus *Homo*, and species Homo sapiens. Why was man placed in this category along with kangaroos, moles, duckbill platypuses, horses, rabbits, bats, and others? Only because this group has three things in common: (1) body temperature is constant, (2) the female has milk glands, and (3) both male and female have hair on their bodies.

It wasn't until the seventeenth century A.D. that an English naturalist named John Ray (1627—1705) attempted to establish a reliable classification system by defining just what a species is. According to Ray, a species is a group of similar individuals having common ancestors. He said, "A species is never born from the seed of another species . . . ."[1] In other words, one species is not produced from another species. John Ray was the first to classify plants and insects into two groups according to species. This method of classification he described in his publications *Methodus Plantarum Nova* (1682), and in *Historia Insectorum*, which was published in 1710, five years after his death.

Our present-day classification system can be traced back to the work of the Swedish botanist Karl von Linné, usually known as Linnaeus (1707—1778), who felt that finding order in nature should be the major aim of science. He believed that every organism had a special place in the scheme of life, and he wanted to classify each organism according to its proper place. Linnaeus's system involved grouping similar species into larger groups known as *genera*. Since Linnaeus's time the original system has many times been reorganized by biologists seeking a more exact classification, but the basic categories of Linnaeus's classification system still remain.

Every living organism is a system of molecules organized in precise patterns. Man is a multicellular organism and an example of an extremely complex, highly organized system of molecules. During the nineteenth century, through the work of the German biologist Theodor Schwann, a statement was issued about the theory of animals and how they functioned. Schwann had been observing animal cells, which led him to the following

[1]American Institute of Biological Sciences, Biological Sciences Curriculum Study, *Biological Science, Molecules to Man* (Boston: Houghton Mifflin Company, 1963), p. 23.

generalization: "The elementary parts of all tissues are formed of cells . . . so that it may be asserted that there is one universal principle of development for the elementary parts of organisms, however different, and that this principle is the formation of cells."[2] Man, the "human machine" is a wonderful, exciting, complex, and always interesting arrangement of cells.

NEW WORDS

Hypotheses (hī-poth'-e-sēs): Tentative theories provisionally adapted to explain certain facts and to guide in the investigation of others.

Homo sapiens (hō'-mō sā'-pi-enz): Mankind.

THE BODY'S STRUCTURAL UNITS

Cells

All living things are made up of cells—from the single-celled amoeba that looks, when highly magnified, like a blob of jelly, to the multicellular organism, man. The individual cell unit is very complex and has many duties. It is like a person living in a bustling metropolis whose citizens are unlike in appearance, who lead very different life styles, but who are similar in that they move, grow, react, protect themselves, and reproduce.

These structural units, or cells, are composed essentially of three main parts: the *membrane*, the *cytoplasm*, and the *nucleus*. There are, however, many other interesting minute structures (too numerous to mention) inside the cell that assist in performing its many specific functions. Although all cells function as living units, they still must depend on one another for life support, much the same as man must depend on others for his life support.

The human body is composed of millions of cells, each performing a specialized function. These cells will vary in size, shape and consistency; but all are composed chiefly of water (90%), plus a small amount of a viscid, translucent colloid material that resembles egg white (protoplasm), and some sugar, starch, fats, and salts.

Man has survived to this point in time because of the effective control of cellular activities within his body and because what began as one cell becomes two and so on until the wonderful machine known as a human is complete. The following list defines the parts of the cell and their individual functions. All these parts are then illustrated in the accompanying diagram on page 5.

Cell Structure	Function
Cell Membrane	This very thin membrane forms the outer wall of all cells and maintains the individuality of cell form. This membrane also controls the exchange of materials between the cell and the environment by osmosis, phagocytosis, pinocytosis, secretion, and other phenomena. It is a very selective, permeable barrier.

[2]Ibid., p. 236.

Cell Structure	Function
Nucleus	The (nu'-kle-us) is the cell brain or control center that contains the chromosomes holding the hereditary material.
Nucleoplasm	The (nu'-kle-ō-plaz-m) is the protoplasm within the nucleus.
Nucleolus	The (nu'-kle-ō-lus) is a fairly large nutlike shape within the nucleus. It is still somewhat of a mystery. However, it is thought to be a vital source of nuclear protein. It is known to be high in RNA (ribonucleic acid). RNA is the messenger that transmits the messages outside the membrane of the nucleus.
Cytoplasm	The (sī'-tō-plaz-m) is a complex, viscous, fluidlike material surrounding the nucleus. It contains the cytoplasmic ribosomes that are the major sites of protein synthesis.
Endoplasmic reticulum	The (en'-do-plas-mic re-tik'-u-lum) is a network of channels extending through the cytoplasm. These channels function as a circulatory system, allowing the ribosomes to transport the proteins they have made.
Ribosomes	The (ri'-bō-sōmes) are small units that look like buckshot scattered along the endoplasmic reticulum. They manufacture protein under the supervision of the nucleus.
Vacuoles	The (vac'-u-ōles) are spaces within the cell; rarely are they found in animal cells.
Centrosome	The (sen'-trō-sōm) is an organelle whose name means "central body." It lies at one side of the nucleus. Within it are two centrioles (sen'-tree-ōls). The centrioles are important during cell division when they duplicate themselves and separate, moving toward opposite sides of the nucleus. Fiberlike rays then develop about each centriole. The cytoplasm is then divided by a furrow that deepens until it completely separates the two new cells. This cell division is called *mitosis* (mī-tō'-sis).
Golgi complex	This structure was named for Camillo Golgi, who first saw it in the brain cells of an owl.[3] It is thought that these small organelles (or"-gah-nels'), which are arranged around the centrosome, make carbohydrate compounds, combine them with certain protein molecules, and then send the package through the cell wall and distribute the contents where needed. There are, however, few scientifically proven facts.
Mitochondria	The (mi"-tō-kon'-dre-ah) are very small rods known as the *powerhouse* of the cell. They are responsible for respiratory and other metabolic functions. They supply the energy that all cells need for life.

[3]George G. Simpson and William S. Beck, *Life: An Introduction to Biology* (New York: Harcourt Brace Jovanovich, Inc., 1965), p. 76.

Cell Structure	Function
Lysosome	The (li′-so-sōme) is an organelle containing chemicals that will digest food compounds, and under certain conditions will destroy microbes by digesting them.
Chromosomes	The (kro′-mo-sōmes) contain all the hereditary information for the reproduction of new cells. The main chemical is the fascinating DNA (de-oxe″-ri″-bo-nu-cle′-ic acid). DNA is the master that issues the orders of life from the nucleus. DNA is sometimes called the "code of life". It is the director. It establishes primary control over the activities and processes of virtually all cells. It is also the source of heriditary instructions.

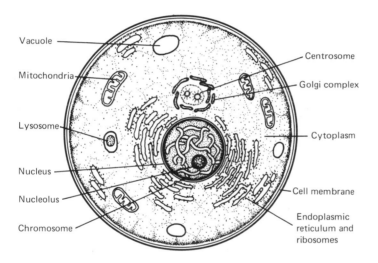

A diagrammatic drawing of a cell and its basic components.

NEW WORDS

Metabolic (met′-a-bol-ik′): Pertaining to processes concerned with the disposition of the nutrients absorbed into the blood following digestion.

Organelle (or″-gàh-nel): A minute structure serving a specific function in the life processes of a cell.

Osmosis (os-mō′-sis): Diffusion of water through a semipermeable membrane.

Permeable (pur′-mē-à-bl): Allowing passage of fluids.

Phagocytosis (fag′-ō-sī-tō′-sis): The uptake or envelopment of solid particles by living cells.

Pinocytosis (pin″-ȯ-sī-tō′-sis): The uptake of fluid material by a living cell, particularly by means of invagination of the cell membrane and by vacuole formation.

Synthesis (sin′-thē-sis): Creation of a compound by union of the elements composing it, either by artificial or natural processes.

Viscous (vis′-kus): Sticky or gummy.

The sequence of cell division (mitosis) is shown in the series of drawings below:

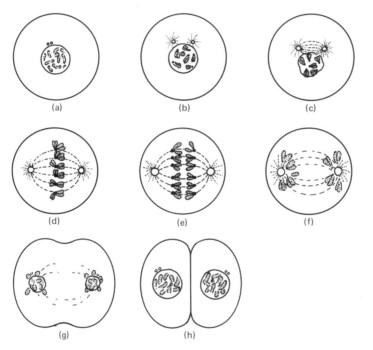

Mitosis. (a) Resting cell with nucleus and centrosome; (b) resting cell with nucleus and centrosomes; (c) centrosomes separating; (d) chromosomes lying in the center; (e) chromosomes divided into halves; (f) chromosomes separating; (g) chromosomes forming two nuclei, and cell body beginning to divide; (h) cell division complete.

SELF—TEST

1. Name the three major parts of the cell. _____

2. Give the percentage of water, and name the five other substances found in cells. _____

3. What controls the exchange of materials between the cell and the envi-

ronment? _____

4. What are the major sites of protein synthesis and where are they located?

_____

5. What is the control center of the cell and explain why it is so called?

_____

6. Name two substances found in the control center, and tell which is called the *director* and which is called the *messenger.* _____

_____

7. What is the importance of the centrosome? _____

8. Explain the meaning of *mitosis.* _____

9. What are the mitochondria, and what do they supply that all cells need for life? _____

_____

10. What important information is supplied by the chromosomes? _____

_____

Tissues and Membranes

Tissues. A tissue may be defined as a group of similar cells forming a particular function but whose appearance and structure vary greatly. Man is composed of a variety of tissues. However, basically these tissues fall into four groups: (1) epithelial, (2) muscle, (3) nerve, and (4) connective. The following section describes the functions of each of these groups of tissues.

Tissue	Function
Epithelial	The (ep″-i-thē-lē-al) tissue is a surface tissue, devoid of blood vessels and nourished by lymph, whose primary function is to protect and repair; however, it is also involved in absorption, secretion, and special sensation. It covers the outer layer of the skin and also some internal surfaces. There are many kinds of epithelial tissue, and the function of each is determined by its location.
	Squamous epithelium occurs as a single layer of cells and is sometimes classed as *simple epithelium.* This type of epithelium lines the air passages of the lungs and also lines the heart and the blood vessels. Another type of squamous epithelium is *stratified* (occurring in several layers). It is found lining invaginations such as the mouth, nose, and anus. The deeper layer of this type of epithelium is composed of cells that are continually multiplying and growing in size, pushing the older cells gradually outward and upward.

Tissue	Function

These older cells grow harder as they near the outer surface. In this manner nature has found a way to replace the outermost surface of cells that is continually being rubbed away. *Columnar epithelial* cells derive their name from the fact that they are set upright in columns on the surface that they cover. This type of tissue is found lining the stomach and portions of the intestines.

Ciliated epithelium is columnar epithelium that is covered with minute hairlike processes that are continually vibrating in a lashing wavelike motion. These hairlike processes are called *cilia*. This tissue is found in parts of the respiratory tract, brain, spinal cord, and reproductive organs.

Sensory epithelium contains the end organs of nerves, such as the olfactory nerve in the nose and the auditory nerve in the epithelium of the middle ear.

Glandular epithelium consists of cells that have accumulated mucoid secretion and have assumed a chalice form.

Connective

Connective tissue varies greatly in form and has many functions. These functions basically are: *supportive*, *binding*, and *specialized*. Connective tissue can develop in any part of the body to repair or replace damaged tissue. This new growth is known as *scar tissue*.

Supportive: This is cartilage or soft connective tissue. It is rubbery in texture, and it is designed to resist compression. This tissue provides the pattern of the human embryo, and it is ultimately resorbed in most areas, as mineral salts in solution are deposited to produce osseous tissue, or hard tissue, which then becomes the human skeleton. In some areas such as joints, segments of the spine, and the ends of long bones, remnants of cartilage may be found. Nature has thus provided a means of reducing friction between moving parts. Some other parts of the human body that are made up of cartilage are the nose, ears, epiglottis, and parts of the larynx.

Binding (loose connective tissue): This tissue binds muscle cells into individual muscles and nerve fibers into individual nerves, as well as binding all kinds of organs in a loose but strong manner. The weaker fibrous connective tissue is found under the epithelium of the skin and the mucous membrane. The stronger fibrous tissue is found in the tendons and ligaments that assist in giving movement to our body. This strength is necessary since tendons must bind muscle to bone so as to allow muscle contraction sufficient to move bone. Ligaments must be tough and elastic; they connect bones at a joint, or support organs, keeping them in place but allowing movement as the body moves.

Specialized (fluid): This tissue comprises the internal fluids such as the blood and the lymph that contain cells but whose intercellular matrix is fluid.

Tissue	Function
Nerve	Nerve tissue is a part of the entire nervous system. It is composed of nerve cells (neurons) and long protoplasmic fibers held together by connective tissue to form nerves. Its function is to transmit information by means of electrical impulses from one nerve cell to another. It is the link between every structure in the body and the body's central control station, the brain. In some areas, nerve tissue is capable of slow repair when injured; but in other areas, no repair is possible.
Muscle	Muscle tissue is fully developed to produce powerful contractions. The cells are long and threadlike, and they may be divided into three categories: (1) skeletal, (2) cardiac, and (3) visceral. Muscle tissue, like nerve tissue, repairs itself with difficulty or not at all; it is frequently replaced with scar tissue. *Skeletal* (striated): This tissue produces body movement, and because it will contract by an act of will, it is called *voluntary*. *Cardiac* (striated): This muscle, although striated, is different from skeletal muscle tissue. This tissue comprises the bulk of the heart wall and is responsible for the beating of the heart. *Visceral* (smooth): This tissue forms the walls of the organs of the ventral body cavities and is responsible for the movement of food along the digestive tract; it makes up the lining of blood vessels and of the tubes carrying urine from the kidneys. It also is found at the base of body hairs.

NEW WORDS

Absorption (ab-sorp'-shun): The act of taking up or in by specific chemical or molecular action.

Chalice (chal'-is): A drinking cup, goblet; especially the cup used in the Sacrament of the Lord's Supper.

Ciliated (sil'-ē-āt"-ed): Provided with cilia (hairlike projections).

Matrix (mā'-triks): That which gives form, origin, or foundation to something. In anatomy and biology, it refers to the intercellular substance of a tissue.

Osseous (os'-sē-us): Composed of or resembling bone.

Protoplasmic (prō'-tō-plaz'-mik): Pertaining to the essential substance of both cell and nucleus; a viscous translucent material that holds fine granules in suspension.

Secretion (se-kre'-shun): The process of elaborating a specific product as a result of the activity of a gland. One example is saliva produced by salivary glands.

Squamous (skwa'-mus): Scaly or platelike.

Membranes. A membrane is a thin layer of tissue that covers a surface or divides an organ. The body membranes may be divided into four classifications: (1) serous, (2) synovial, (3) mucous, and (4) cutaneous. The functions of the four classes of membranes are given below.

Membrane	Function
Serous	The serous membranes are thin, transparent, fairly strong, and elastic. They derive their name from the serum (fluid) moistening their surfaces. These membranes line the closed cavities and passages that *do not communicate with the exterior*. One example would be the pericardium, which covers the heart. The most important function of these membranes is protection.
Synovial	The synovial membranes are sometimes classed as serous membranes because their function and location are much the same; however, in secretion and structure they are different. They are associated with the bones and muscles rather than with the viscera. They are thin, delicate connective tissues that secrete a viscid fluid resembling egg white. One example would be the membrane surrounding and lubricating the cavities of a movable joint, such as the temperomandibular joint that allows articulation between the mandible and the temporal bone of the skull.
Mucous	The mucous membranes line passages and cavities that *communicate with the exterior*. Their surfaces are coated with mucous, and they are divided into two groups: (1) the *gastropulmonary* (gas"-trō-pul'-mo-ner"-e) mucous membrane, which commences at the lips and nostrils and continues the entire length of the alimentary canal to the anus; and (2) the *genitourinary* (jen"-i-to-u'-ri-ner"-e) mucous membrane, which lines the inside of the bladder and the whole of the urinary tract. In the female this membrane also lines the vagina, uterus, and the Fallopian tubes. The mucous membranes are composed of epithelial tissue as well as connective tissue containing blood vessels. There is also a thin layer of muscular tissue that allows cavities such as the esophagus to expand during swallowing. The main function of these mucous membranes are: protection, support of blood vessels and lymphatics, and provision of large surfaces for absorption and secretion of mucus.
Cutaneous	This membrane consists of two layers: (1) the *epidermis*, and (2) the *corum* (a highly sensitive vascular layer of connective tissue). The cutaneous membrane is the outer

Membrane	Function
Cutaneous (continued)	layer, or skin, that protects deeper tissues, regulates body heat, contains sense organs, and acts as an excretory and respiratory organ.

NEW WORDS

Pericardium (per″-i-kar′-dē-um): The fibroserous sac that surrounds the heart, comprising an external layer of dense fibrous tissue and an inner serous layer.

Temperomandibular (tem″-po-ro-man″-dib-u′-lar): Pertaining to joining of the mandible to the temporal bone of the skull.

SELF—TEST

1. Where is epithelial tissue found, and what are its chief functions? _____

_____

2. What is ciliated epithelial tissue? _____

3. Define secretion. _____

4. Define absorption. _____

5. Name three basic functions of connective tissue. _____

_____

6. Where is cartilage found? What is its texture and function? _____

_____

7. Tendons and ligaments are types of connective tissue. What are their function(s)? _____

_____

8. Are blood and lymph considered tissues? _____

9. Muscle tissue has three groupings; name them and give the function of each. _____

_____

10. What is the function of nerve tissue? _____

11. Where are serous membranes found, and what is their most important function? _____

_____

12. Where are synovial membranes found? _____

13. Where are mucous membranes found, and what are their main functions?

_____

14. Are mucous membranes composed of epithelium and connective tissue?

_____

15. What is the cutaneous membrane? Give its functions. _____

_____

THE BODY'S LANDMARKS

To understand directions, it is important that the reader be acquainted with certain body landmarks and the terminology used to locate various organs. The body is like a map; and, like a map, landmarks are very necessary when exploring in order not to become lost. This information and the information in the following pages will give some terms, positions, and landmarks that will assist the reader when studying the body systems.

Body Cavities

Dorsal Cavity. The dorsal cavity includes the _cranial_ and the _spinal_ subcavities, which in turn contain the brain and the spinal cord.

Ventral Cavity. The ventral cavity contains three subcavities: (1) the _thoracic_ cavity, which contains the trachea, lungs, esophagus, heart, and the great vessels springing from and entering into the heart; (2) the _abdominal_ cavity, which contains the stomach, liver, gallbladder, pancreas, spleen, and small and large intestines; and (3) the _pelvic_ cavity, which contains the bladder, rectum, and some reproductive organs. The diaphragm forms a muscularfibrous partition between the thoracic and abdominal cavities.

In some cases those cavities with external openings such as the _orbital_ cavity, which contains the eye, optic nerve, muscles of the eyeball, and the lacrimal apparatus; the _nasal_ cavity, which includes the structures that form the nose; and the _oral_ cavity, which contains the tongue, teeth, and salivary glands, are also listed as body cavities.

The figure on page 13 illustrates the main body cavities.

Terminology

Some of the directional terms listed below are illustrated by a diagrammatic drawing on the next page.

Body Landmark	Definition
Anterior	Situated in front of.
Caudal	Pertaining to the distal end of the body.
Cephalic	Pertaining to the head end of the body.
Cranial	Pertaining to the cranium, or to the anterior (front) or superior end of the body.

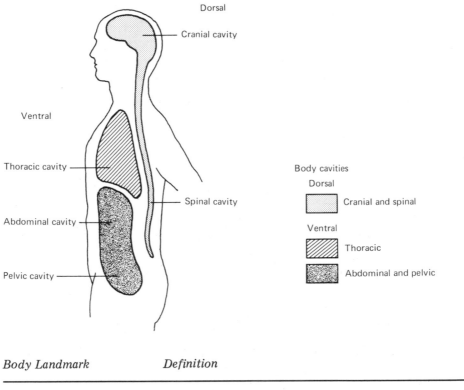

Body Landmark	Definition
Deep	Extending far below the surface.
Distal	Away from the median line (farthest away from the point of attachment.)
Dorsal	Of or near the back; behind. Also pertaining to the top of the foot, or the back of the hand. Used the same as "posterior."
External	Outer.
Frontal plane	A vertical plane passing longitudinally through the body from side to side at right angles to the median plane that divides the body into front and back.
Inferior	Below, or toward the tail end of the body. Used the same as "caudal."
Internal	Inner, the same as "deep."
Lateral	To the side.
Medial	Toward the median line; also called midline.
Median plane	A longitudinal plane that divides the body into right and left halves (from front to back).
Palmar	Of, in, or corresponding to the palm of the hand.
Plantar	Of or on the sole of the foot.
Posterior	Situated in back of.

Body Landmark	Definition
Proximal	Nearest to the point of attachment, or nearest the center of the body.
Sagittal plane	Any plane parallel to the median plane dividing the body into right and left positions.
Superficial	On or near the surface.
Superior	Situated above.
Transverse plane	The horizontal plane. A section at right angles to the frontal plane.
Ventral	At or toward the front of the body; toward the belly.

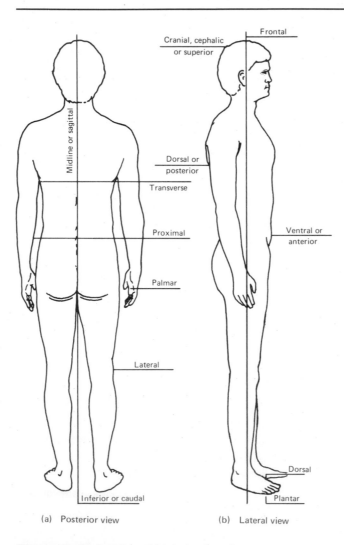

(a) Posterior view   (b) Lateral view

Diagrammatic drawing of body landmarks.

SELF—TEST

1. Name the cavities where the following are found.

   (a) Brain. _____

   (b) Rectum. _____

   (c) Heart. _____

   (d) Lungs. _____

   (e) Reproductive organs. _____

   (f) Intestines. _____

   (g) Bladder. _____

   (h) Spinal Cord. _____

   (i) Liver. _____

2. Turn to page 16 and fill in the body landmark terms on the blank lines provided.

THE BODY'S SYSTEMS

The Reproductive System

Only through sexual reproduction are human beings immortal. It is known that life comes only from other life and that a human being, a most complex organism, does not arise by chance but by the sperm of the male fertilizing the egg cell, or *ovum*, of the female. This is sexual reproduction. This fertilized ovum or one-celled embryo is called a *zygote* (zi'-gōt). After fertilization, the zygote divides and subdivides until many cells form a three-layered membrane known as the *blastoderm*. The three layers are individually known as the *ectoderm* (outer layer), the *mesoderm* (middle layer), and the *entoderm* (inner layer). The human body as we know it, ultimately develops entirely from these three embryonic layers.

This concept of reproduction was not always considered correct. During the latter part of the seventeenth and early part of the eighteenth centuries, much controversy existed as to how man developed. One school of thought asserted that in the egg cell there existed a preformed human being and the sperm was only necessary to trigger growth of the preformed human. Another school of thought claimed that the preformed adult lay in the sperm head.[4] We now know that what begins as one cell is first fertilized by sperm and then divides, differentiates, and ultimately becomes the multicellular being known as man.

The following section lists the functions and location of female and male organs.

[4]George G. Simpson and William S. Beck. *Life: An Introduction to Biology* 2nd ed. (New York: Harcourt Brace Jovanovich, Inc., 1965), p. 43.

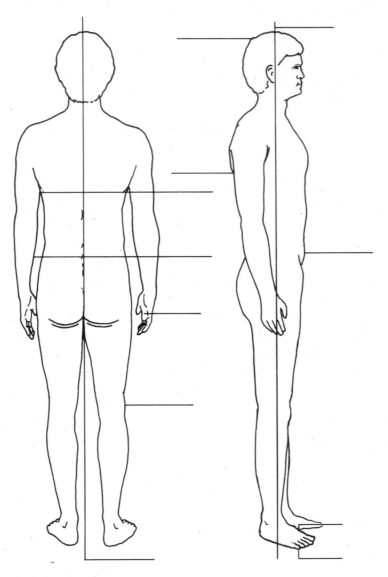

Body Landmarks.

Female Organs	Location and Function
Vagina	The (vah-ji′-nuh) is the sexual canal of the female. It is also the birth canal. It lies in the pelvic cavity behind the bladder and in front of the rectum. It extends to the uterus. The sperm of the male enters the vagina and travels to the uterine tubes, via the canal and the uterus, to meet the ovum.
Ovaries	The ovaries are the sex glands (female gonads) in which ova (egg cells) are produced. These glands are located on either

Female Organs	*Location and Function*
Ovaries (continued)	side of the uterus and deep within the pelvic area of the abdomen. The hormones secreted by the ovaries are: (1) *estrogen*, which plays a part in the development of the reproductive organs and sex characteristics of the female; and (2) *progesterone*, which plays a part in the menstrual cycle and assists in preparing the uterus for possible conception.
Follicle	The (fol'-i-cl) is a tiny saclike structure within the ovary that contains the developing egg. The follicle grows and becomes filled with fluid; and when the egg is ripe and almost ready for fertilization, the follicle ruptures near the surface of the ovary. The egg is then carried out with the fluid, through the uterine tube, toward the uterus. This is called *ovulation* (ō''-vu-lā'-shun). This release of the egg cell occurs about once in every 28 days.
Oviduct	After the egg leaves the ovary, it enters the (oh'-vih-dukt), also known as a *Fallopian tube* or *uterine tube*, where fertilization either does or does not take place. If fertilization takes place, the egg continues through the oviduct and enters the uterus, where it normally lodges and begins to develop.
Uterus	The (yew'-ter-us) is also known as the *womb*. It is a thick-walled, hollow, muscular organ situated in the pelvis between the bladder and the rectum. This organ prepares to receive the mature egg each month. Eggs that are not fertilized are eliminated during the menses. When this occurs, the monthly cycle begins again. Further development of the embryo is a very complex process and will not be discussed in this text, with the exception of a brief description of the development of the head and neck in Chapter 2.

Male Organs	*Location and Function*
Penis	The penis is the external organ for urination and for introduction of sperm cells into the female vagina.
Scrotum	The (skrō'-tum) is a skin-covered pouch that contains the testes and accessory organs.
Testes	The testes (also called the *testicles*) are oval-shaped glands that form millions of male sex cells known as *sperm* or *spermatozoa*. These sex cells, upon joining within the uterine tube with the female ovum, eventually become another human being. The hormone that is secreted by the testes is called *testosterone* (tes-tos'-te-rōn). It stimulates male reproductive organs, and plays a part in sex characteristics such as beard growth, muscle strength, etc.

Male Organs	Location and Function
Epididymide	The (ep″-i-did′-i-mid-e) is a long, narrow tubule lying along the upper posterior border of the testicles. It is lined with mucous membrane and serves as a storage place for sperm.
Vas deferens	The vas deferens is the continuation of the epididymides. Sperm produced in the testes depart from the body via the epididymides to the vas deferens where they are ejaculated deep into the female vagina.

SELF—TEST

1. Name the three embryonic layers of the blastoderm. ―――――――

―――――――――――――――――――――――――

2. Does the entire human body develop from these three layers? ―――――

3. Name the five main parts of the female sex organs. ―――――――

―――――――――――――――――――――――――

4. Which glands are known as the *female gonads*? ―――――――

5. Which glands produce the egg cells? ―――――――

6. Name the five male sex organs. ―――――――

7. What female organs secrete hormones, and what are the names of those hormones? ―――――――

8. What male sex organs secrete a hormone, and what is the name of that hormone? ―――――――

9. Define *ovulation*. ―――――――

10. Define *menses*. ―――――――

The Skeletal System

For building anything from a car to a skyscraper there has to be a plan and a blueprint, including such things as the framework, external covering, internal wiring, plumbing, communication systems, etc., all added together to complete the project. When conception takes place, the chromosomes draw the blueprint of the human body and dictate the plan; and, as with other projects, things sometimes do not go exactly according to the blueprint, but, generally, all goes well. The framework of the human body is the skeleton, which is composed of bones and joints put together in such a manner as to complete the general size, shape, and outline designed by the chromosomes. Other body systems take care of the rest of the plan.

Bone, the building material of the skeleton, is connective tissue filled with a variety of living bone cells (osteoblasts, osteoclasts, osteocytes) and blood vessels. The bone cells are surrounded by and embedded in a matrix of nonliving substance. These bone cells are not isolated, however, because a series of canals (canaliculi) run through the matrix allowing movement to some of the cells. Bone is noted for its high mineral content (calcium and phosphorous); and as there is a continuous loss of these minerals through the kidneys and digestive tract, and since cells of the body tissues other than bone also require these minerals, the minerals must be constantly replaced. If these minerals are not in sufficient quantity in the diet, they will be withdrawn from the skeleton, leaving, as in the case of starvation, bone that is soft and spongy. During pregnancy the mother's body must supply the infant's body with materials for its skeleton. Therefore, expectant mothers frequently supplement their diets with calcium tablets. Hormones also play a part in the control of bone formation. This will be discussed later.

Bone is composed of several layers of tissue with many nerves and blood vessels in all layers. The outer layer is called the *periosteum*. It is a tough but thin membrane that supports tendons and serves as a protection. It encloses all bones except at the joints. Directly under the periosteum is the *compact bone*. It is a dense, hard fibrous tissue. The *cancellous bone* then comes immediately under the compact bone. It is filled with spaces giving it a spongy appearance.

The *marrow* occupies the center of the bone; it contains a network of blood vessels and connective tissue holding the cells together. The cells manufactured in the red bone marrow are erythrocytes, leukocytes, and platelets. During infancy and childhood all bone marrow is red. However as one grows older, in some bones the marrow turns yellow and no longer is capable of producing cells except in cases of extreme emergency.

Skeletal bones are divided into 2 main groups (1) the axial and (2) the appendicular. In all, there are 206 bones of various sizes and shapes in the human skeleton. The following section provides a brief description of the major skeletal bones in each of the two main groups: axial and appendicular.

A detailed discussion of the bones of the head (cranial and facial) will be covered in Chapter 2.

Axial Bones

Bone	Description
Vertebrae	There are 33 vertebrae in a child's vertebral column and 26 in an adult vertebral column. This apparent decrease is due to the union, in the adult, of the sacral bones and the coccyx (kok'-sics) bones. There are 5 sections in the vertebral column; these are: (1) cervical, (2) thoracic, (3) lumbar, (4) sacral, and (5) coccygeal (kok-si-j'-e-al). *Cervical*: The cervical bones are located in the neck and are 7 in number. The first vertebra, or *atlas*, supports the head. It was named after the Greek god who bears up the pillars of heaven. The second vertebra, or *axis*, contains the process that forms a pivot around which the atlas rotates when the head is turned.

Bone	Location and Description
Vertebrae (continued)	*Thoracic:* The 12 thoracic vertebrae form the posterior wall of the thorax or chest. They give attachment to the ribs. *Lumbar:* The 5 lumbar vertebrae are located between the thoracic vertebrae and the sacrum. They are the largest and heaviest of the vertebrae. *Sacral:* Also called the *sacrum.* Dorsally and between the 2 hip bones are the 5 fused sacral vertebrae forming one large triangular bone. These vertebrae are known as *false vertebrae.* *Coccygeal:* The coccyx is usually formed from 3 to 5 small segments of bone. It is below the sacrum and it is the most underdeveloped part of the vertebral column.
Skull	The skull consists of the 22 cranial and facial bones; these will be discussed in detail in Chapter 2.
Thorax	The thorax or the thoracic cavity is formed anteriorly by the sternum and the costal cartilages (the cartilage between the true ribs and the sternum), with 12 ribs on each side; and posteriorly by the bodies of the 12 thoracic vertebrae. The thorax supports the bones of the shoulder girdle and upper extremities. It contains and protects the principal organs of respiration and circulation.
Sternum	The sternum (breast bone) is a narrow flat plate of bone about 6 inches long and is situated anteriorly on the median line of the chest. It develops as three parts: the upper part or handle, the middle or body, and the inferior or xiphoid (zif'-oid) process. Seven costal cartilages are attached to the upper and middle pieces. The xiphoid, or lower part, has no ribs attached but does afford attachment for some abdominal muscles. Care must be taken not to break this process when giving cardiopulmonary resuscitation.
Ribs	There are a total of 24 ribs. There are 12 on either side of the thoracic cavity. All 24 ribs are connected dorsally to the vertebrae. The first 7 are attached anteriorly to the sternum and are called the *true ribs.* The remaining 5 are termed *false ribs.* Of these 5 false ribs, 8, 9, and 10 are attached anteriorly to the costal cartilages of the rib immediately above. The 2 lowest are attached only to the vertebrae and are called *floating ribs.*

Appendicular Bones: Upper Extremities and Attachments

Bone	Description
Clavicle	The (clav'-i-cle), also called the *collar bone,* is a long slender bone placed horizontally above the thorax. It is attached medially to the sternum and laterally to the scapula.

Bone	Description
Scapula	The (skap′-ū-la) is another name for the *shoulder blade*. It is a large, flat triangular bone in the back of the shoulder.
Humerus	The (hū′-mer-us) is the longest bone in the upper arm. It extends from the shoulder to the elbow.
Ulna	The (ul′-na) is the larger bone of the forearm. It is placed at the inner, or little finger side, and lies parallel to the radius.
Radius	The (rā′-dĭ-us) is the small outer bone of the forearm.
Carpus	The (kär′-pus), or wrist, consists of 8 small bones, the carpals, which are united by ligaments so arranged as to allow some motion.
Metacarpus	The (met′-a-kär′-pus) is formed by 5 bones, the metacarpals. It is the hand.
Phalanges	The (fal′-an-jēz) are the bones of the fingers. There are 14 in each hand with 3 in each finger and 2 in the thumb. There are a total of 27 bones in the hand and wrist.

Appendicular Bones: Lower Extremities and Attachments

Bone	Description
Hip bones	The innominate or hip bones are 2 large irregularly shaped bones that form the sides and front wall of the pelvic cavity. Although each is fused into only one bone in the adult, each one is made up of three portions: the illium, ischium, and pubis. *Illium* (il′-ē-um): The lateral flaring portion that forms the prominence of the hip bone. *Ischium* (is′-kē-um): The inferior, dorsal, and strongest portion of the hip bone. *Pubis* (pū′-bis): Anterior portion of the hip bone, also called the *pubic bone*.
Pelvis	So named as it resembles a basin. It is composed of 4 bones: 2 hip bones, the sacrum, and the coccyx.
Femur	The (fē′-mer) is the thigh bone. It extends from the pelvis to the knee. It is the longest and strongest bone in the skeleton.
Patella	The (pa-tel′-a) is the knee cap. It is a small, thick, flat, movable triangular bone that is situated anteriorly at the knee joint.
Tibia	The (tib′-i-a) is the shin bone. It is the larger inner bone of the leg below the knee.
Fibula	The (fib′-ū-la) is the lateral and smaller of the 2 leg bones. It is the most slender of the long bones. It lies parallel with the tibia.

Bone	Description
Tarsus	The (tar'-sus) is the ankle; it is composed of 7 small tarsal bones. The largest of these 7 bones is the heel bone. The tarsus forms the articulation between the foot and the leg.
Metatarsus	The metatarsus is the sole or the instep. There are 5 metatarsal bones that resemble the metacarpal bones of the hand.
Phalanges	The phalanges also resemble the bones in the hand in that there are 3 phalanges in the toes and 2 in the great (big) toe.

NEW WORDS

Cardiopulmonary resuscitation: Another name for heart-lung resuscitation, or the combination of efforts to restore breathing and circulation artificially.

Erythrocytes (ē-rith'-rō-sīts): Red blood cells or corpuscles. These are the principal carriers of oxygen to all parts of the body.

Leukocytes (lu'-kō-sītes"): White blood cells. They protect the body against disease-causing microorganisms.

Osteocytes (os'-te-o-sīts"): Cells lodged in bone that communicate with other cytoplasmic processes. They assist in developing bone.

Osteoblasts (os'-te-ō-blasts"): Immature bone-producing cells.

Platelets: Small disks in the blood that assist in coagulation.

Study the illustration on page 23 that locates the axial and appendicular bones. Then take the self tests on pages 24 and 25.

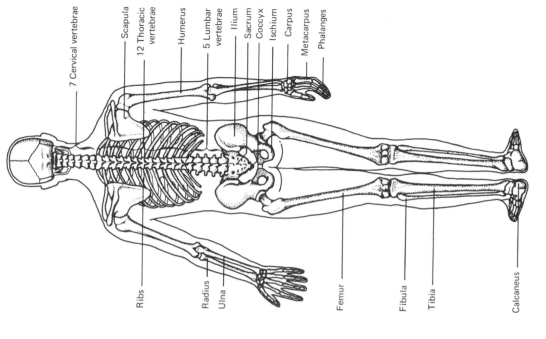

7 Cervical vertebrae

Scapula

12 Thoracic vertebrae

Humerus

5 Lumbar vertebrae

Ilium

Sacrum

Coccyx

Ischium

Carpus

Metacarpus

Phalanges

Ribs

Radius

Ulna

Femur

Fibula

Tibia

Calcaneus

(b) Skeleton Posterior View

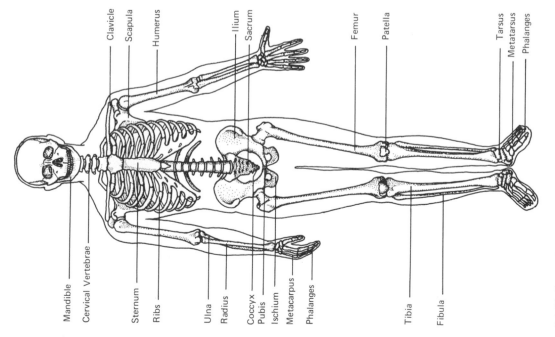

Clavicle

Scapula

Humerus

Ilium

Sacrum

Femur

Patella

Tarsus

Metatarsus

Phalanges

Mandible

Cervical Vertebrae

Sternum

Ribs

Ulna

Radius

Coccyx

Pubis

Ischium

Metacarpus

Phalanges

Tibia

Fibula

(a) Skeleton Anterior View

SELF—TEST

1. Define the following:

 (a) Periosteum. _____

 (b) Erythrocytes. _____

 (c) Compact bone. _____

 (d) Cancellous bone. _____

 (e) Marrow. _____

 (f) Canaliculi. _____

 (g) Osteoblasts. _____

 (h) Leukocytes. _____

 (i) Platelets. _____

2. Into what two main groups are skeleton bones divided? _____

3. How many vertebrae does an adult have? _____

4. The vertebrae are divided into five sections. Please name these sections and give the number of vertebrae in each. _____
_____

5. Where is the xiphoid process located? _____

6. How many ribs are there? _____

7. Which ribs are called *floating ribs*? _____

8. Locate the bones of the skeleton on the skematic drawing on the next page. Write in the names of the axial and appendicular bones.

The Nervous System

The body systems do not function individually; they are an integrated system of checks and balances, with the nervous system acting as the coordinator for all. The body's internal reactions to stimuli and its adjustments to the environment are controlled by the nervous system. Night and day, a brain weighing approximately 3 pounds, with over 12 billion nerve cells, sends out electrical impulses at a speed of about 100 meters per second. This is accomplished by bundles of nerves that may contain, in each bundle, as many as 25,000 nerve fibers. Should the nervous system collapse, utter chaos would result.

The nervous system is separated into two large divisions: (1) the *central nervous system* and (2) the *peripheral nervous system* and the autonomic nervous system, which is not an independent system but a part of the pre-

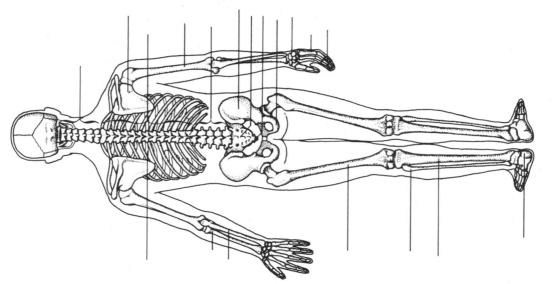

(b) Skeleton Posterior View

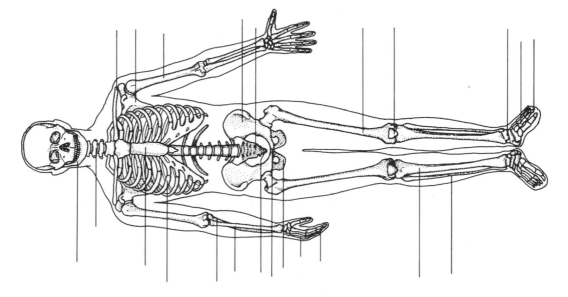

(a) Skeleton Anterior View

25

ceding systems. The central nervous system and the 12 cranial nerves that are part of the peripheral nervous system will be briefly discussed. The fifth cranial nerve, or the *trigeminal nerve*, which is sometimes known as the "dental nerve," will be covered in detail in Chapter 2.

The following describes the nerve cell (neuron), the nerve cell parts, and their functions, as well as the functions of the central and peripheral nervous systems.

Nerve Cell (Neuron)	*Description*
Cell body (cyton)	The cell body or *cyton* of a typical neuron consists of cytoplasm surrounding a large nucleus. Extending from the nerve cell body are two processes (threadlike fibers that carry messages to and from the brain and along the spinal cord).
Dendrites	The dendrites make up the shorter branches of the neuron's two processes; the dendrites are the *afferent* processes or *sensory receptors* that *carry impulses to* the cell body. They vary greatly in size, shape, and number.
Axon	The axon is the longer of the neuron's two processes; it may be as long as 3 feet. This is the *efferent* or *motor effector* fiber that *carries impulses away* from the cell body. Unlike the multiple dendrites, the axon is single. However, there may be a few extensions (collaterals) from the main fiber.

Nerve Parts	*Description*
Nerve	A nerve is a bundle of neurons bound together by connective tissue.
Synapse	A synapse (sin'-aps) is a microscopic gap at the point of contact between two neurons where an impulse is transmitted. It is thought to be a form of control to either speed up or retard the nerve impulses as they travel from one neuron to another.
Nerve impulses	When the end of a nerve fiber is stimulated, the stimulus starts chemical changes and electrical impulses that travel the length of the fiber from the receptor to the effector. These impulses always travel in the same direction.
Receptors	Information about the external world is received through the dendrites, or sensory neurons, which end in receptor cells especially designed to receive stimuli. Each receptor or group of similar receptors is specialized to receive a specific type of stimulus.
Effector	The effector is a motor neuron in which the efferent process (axon) ends in a muscle or gland. When an impulse is conducted to a muscle fiber, it reacts, and this is known as a *reflex arc*.

Central Nervous System (CNS). The CNS consists of the brain and the spinal cord. It is also known as the *voluntary system*. The brain is a large expanded part of the spinal cord occupying the cranial cavity. It is composed of millions of neurons connected with each other and forming a master control network for most bodily functions. It consists of five parts: the cerebrum, cerebellum, midbrain, pons, and the medulla oblongata.

Parts of the Brain	*Description*
Cerebrum	The cerebrum is the largest part of the brain; it is composed of, among other things, grey matter called the cortex (outer layer). The cortex is the thinking/reasoning part of the brain. White matter lies underneath the cortex, and it consists of small fibers that run in three directions to link the different parts of the brain together and to connect the brain with the spinal cord. The cerebrum is covered with fissures, sulci (grooves), and winding folds (convolutions). The cerebrum is divided lengthwise into two hemispheres (halves) by a large fissure called the longitudinal fissure. There is also a transverse fissure between the cerebrum and the cerebellum. The three remaining fissures divide each hemisphere into lobes, the frontal, parietal, temporal, and occipital, named for the bones of the cranium under which they lie. The functions of the cerebrum are: (1) to govern mental activities, (2) to instigate voluntary acts, and (3) to control many reflex acts.
Midbrain	The midbrain is the short part of the brain stem. It lies just above the pons and serves to connect the medulla oblongata, pons, and the cerebellum with the cerebrum.
Pons	The pons lies in front of the cerebellum between the midbrain and the medulla. It unites the two halves of the cerebellum.
Medulla oblongata	The medulla oblongata (spinal bulb) is continuous with the spinal cord. On passing into the cranial cavity through a large opening called the *foramen magnum*, it widens into a pyramidal-shaped mass. A vital part of the brain, the medulla functions as a connecting bridge to allow impulses from most of the nerves to enter and leave the CNS. It is also the control center of many vital body functions, such as blood pressure, heart beat, and respiration. For some reason, the great trunk nerve fibers extending from the brain into the cord and from the cord into the brain cross over in the medulla; because of this, nerves arising in the cortex of the right side of the brain govern the movements of the left side of the body and vice versa.

Spinal Cord. The spinal cord is that part of the central nervous system that lies within the spinal canal. It extends from the foramen magnum, or the occipital bone of the skull, to about the first or second lumbar vertebra, and then it tapers off. The average length is 18 inches. The spinal cord is an important center of reflex action, and it contains the principal conducting pathways for sensory impulses to the brain and motor impulses from the brain.

Peripheral Nervous System (PNS). The PNS consists of the cranial nerves and the ganglia outside the brain and the spinal cord. The 12 cranial nerves and the 31 spinal nerves make up this system. There are 12 pairs of nerves that emerge from the brain. These are known as the *cranial nerves*, deriving their names from their location on the brain. Ten of these 13 nerves supply nerve fibers to the head. One of the 12 extends to muscles in the neck and shoulder, and one nerve branches into the thoracic and abdominal cavity. There are three varieties of nerve fibers in these cranial nerves: (1) afferent, (2) efferent, and (3) mixed (containing both motor and sensory fibers). After these nerve fibers leave the cranium, they split into branches, which are then widely distributed. The location, on the brain, of the 12 nerves is as follows: I through IV are located near the front of the brain; V through VIII are related to the pons, IX through XII are related to the medulla. The individual functions of the 12 cranial nerves are listed below.

Cranial Nerves	Function
I. Olfactory	The (ol-fac'-to-re) nerve is responsible for the sense of smell.
II. Optic	The optic nerve is responsible for the sense of vision.
III. Oculomotor	The (ok″-u-lo-mō'-tor) nerve permits the eye to open and close. It also allows the eyeball to move.
IV. Trochlear	The (trok'-lē-ar) nerve supplies motion to the eyeball.
V. Trigeminal	The (tri-jem'-i-nal) nerve supplies the teeth and muscles of mastication, the anterior portion of the scalp, the eyelids, and the mucosa of the sinus. It has three branches: (1) ophthalmic, (2) maxillary, and (3) mandibular.
VI. Abducens	The (ab-du'-senz) nerve permits motion of the eyeball muscles.
VII. Facial	The facial nerve is largely a motor nerve. It supplies sensation to parts of the muscles of the face and scalp, and to the anterior two-thirds of the tongue; it also stimulates the secretory fibers of the submaxillary and sublingual glands and the vasodilator fibers of the blood vessels of these glands.
VIII. Acoustic	The (ah-koos'-tik) nerve provides a sense of hearing, position, and movement (equilibrium).
IX. Glossopharyngeal	The (glos″-ō-fah-rin'-jē-al) nerve provides sensation to the tongue and pharynx, and reflex action for the heart and swallowing. It stimulates secretions of the parotid glands.

Cranial Nerves	Function
X. Vagus	The vagus nerve is both motor and sensory. It is the longest of the cranial nerves. It supplies the throat, larynx, and most of the organs in the thoracic and abdominal cavities.
XI. Accessory	The accessory nerve is both cranial and spinal. It controls the muscles of the neck and shoulders.
XII. Hypoglossal	The (hi″-pō-glos′-al) nerve is a motor nerve supplying the tongue.

Spinal Nerves. There are 31 spinal nerves. They are named for the regions of the vertebral column from which they emerge, such as L 1 representing the first segment of the lumbar part of the spinal cord, L 2 representing the second segment, etc. These nerves contain both sensory and motor fibers. They continue only a short distance from the spinal cord before branching to supply many parts of the body.

Autonomic Nervous System (ANS). The autonomic nervous system includes certain peripheral nerves with special functions. These functions involve regulating the action of the smooth muscle tissue such as the heart, glands, digestive system, respiratory system, and the skin. This system is also known as the *involuntary system* because it functions without the control of the will.

Sympathetic Nervous System. The sympathetic nervous system is part of the autonomic system; it correlates the activities in widely separated parts of the body. It begins in the spinal cord and extends to the glands and the involuntary muscle tissue. It works with the parasympathetic nervous system.

Parasympathetic Nervous System. The parasympathetic nervous system is also part of the autonomic nervous system. It works with the sympathetic nervous system to keep the body functioning at a near constant rate. An example is the sympathetic system speeding the heart rate and slowing the digestion, while the parasympathetic system does just the opposite.

The Lobes of the Brain. There are four lobes in the brain, and each is responsible for certain vital functions, as noted in the following list.

Lobe	Description
Frontal lobe	This lobe contains the motor cortex that controls the voluntary muscles. It also contains two areas used in speech.
Parietal lobe	This lobe occupies the upper part of each hemisphere; it contains the sensory area in which the general senses such as pain, touch, and temperature are located. Also located in the parietal lobe are such areas as determination of distance, size, and shape.

Lobe	Description
Temporal lobe	This lobe contains the auditory center.
Occipital lobe	This lobe contains the visual area.

The illustration below locates the major parts of the brain and brain stem.

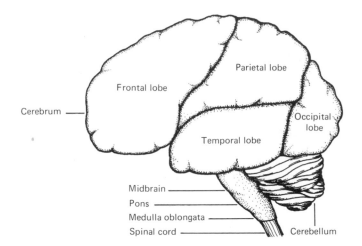

Longitudinal section of the brain locating the four lobes, cerebrum, midbrain, pons, medulla oblongata, spinal cord, and the cerebrum.

SELF—TEST

1. Name the three parts of a neuron._____

2. Which part is afferent and which is efferent? _____

3. Define *afferent* and *efferent*. _____

4. What does CNS stand for and of what does it consist? _____

5. How many cranial nerves are there? _____

6. Which is sometimes known as the "dental nerve"? _____

7. How many spinal nerves are there? _____

8. How are the spinal nerves named? _____

9. Define *autonomic nervous system*. _____

10. Name the two systems that work with the autonomic nervous system.

One of the important functions of the human body is motion. Although there are many types of movement, all types are dependent on the contraction and relaxation of muscular tissue. This tissue is, therefore, classified as *motor tissue*. However, this muscular tissue cannot function alone; it is dependent on the skeletal and nervous systems. All three systems must work together. Improper functioning of any one of the three systems will lessen the usefulness of the others.

There are hundreds of muscles in the human body. Some of the muscles of the trunk and of the upper and lower extremeties will be discussed briefly in this section. Those muscles that are most important to the dental auxiliary will be discussed in more detail in Chapter 2.

There are three characteristics of muscular tissue:

1. *Excitability*: The power to receive and respond quickly to stimuli, thereby causing muscular tissue to contract.
2. *Contractility*: The ability of muscles to change shape.
3. *Extensibility*: The elasticity that gives muscular tissue the ability to stretch.

There are two classifications of movement of muscular tissue:

1. *Voluntary*: Intentional movements that are controlled by the conscious part of the brain or one's own will.
2. *Involuntary*: Movements that are the automatic action of a muscle responding to nerve impulses.

The majority of the sketetal muscles occur in pairs and are usually arranged so that one group opposes the other, resulting in smooth movement. When stimulated, either group of muscles must overcome the resistance of the opposing group in order that contraction takes place more slowly and evenly; smoothness of movement is the result.

Muscle tone means the constant tendency of muscles to contract. This tone is maintained by constant stimuli from the nervous system, stimuli mild enough to maintain firmness but not strong enough to cause motion.

Skeletal muscles, as a rule, contract quickly and relax promptly. However, this might vary according to strength of stimuli, duration of contraction, quality of muscle substance, and temperature. When a muscle receives a series of repeated stimuli so rapidly that there are no periods of relaxation, it loses its excitability from fatigue, causing what is known as *compound contraction* or *tetany* (tet'-an-ne), which is a muscle spasm or cramp.

Muscle tissues are well supplied with blood vessels; and although these blood vessels do not penetrate the cells, each muscle cell is liberally bathed in lymph, which delivers to the cell the materials it needs to maintain its functional activity. The lymph also returns to the blood, waste and materials that can be used by other tissues.

One substance brought to the muscles by the blood is glucose, which is stored in the cells as glycogen. This glycogen represents chemical energy, which may be transformed into mechanical energy when stimulated, allowing muscles to do more work. Waste produced by this action must be eliminated. If these wastes are not eliminated and nutritive materials are lost, prolonged contraction and muscle fatigue will result. Rest, however, will allow the blood to carry waste to the excretory organs and also will allow the blood to bring nutritive materials from the digestive organs to revitalize the fatigued muscles.

The following list gives the form, location, and function of some of the muscles of the body.

Muscle	*Location and Function*
Trapezius[5]	The (trah-pe'-ze-us) muscle is a flat triangular muscle covering the upper and back part of the shoulders, and sloping up toward the base of the skull. It provides movement to the scapula and the head as well as abduction and flexion of the arms.
Sternocleidomastoid	The (ster-no-kli'-do-mas'-toid) is the most prominent muscle of the neck. It forms a cordlike prominence on either side of the neck. It rotates the head and provides lateral movement, turning the face to the opposite side. It gives forward direction to the head when both muscles work together. It also elevates the chin. This muscle arises from the sternum and the clavicle and inserts into the lateral surface of the mastoid process.
Platysma	The (plah-tiz'-mah) is a broad sheet muscle that arises from the skin and the pectoral and deltoid muscles. It inserts in the mandible and the muscles at the angle of the mouth. It depresses the mandible and the lower lip.
Pectoralis major	The (pek"-to-ra'-lis) major is a thick fan-shaped muscle on the ventral and superior part of the chest. It flexes the arm across the chest.
Pectoralis minor	The pectoralis minor is a thin triangular muscle on the cranial part of the thorax and under the pectoralis major. It depresses the shoulder and rotates the scapula downward. It helps to draw the ribs up and expand the chest.
Deltoid	The deltoid is a coarse triangular muscle that covers the shoulder joint ventrally, dorsally, and laterally. This muscle raises the arm to the side, forward, and backward.
Latissimus dorsi	The (lah-tis'-i-mus) dorsi covers the lumbar and the lower half of the posterior thoracic region. It extends, adducts, and rotates the arms medially, and it draws the shoulders down and back.

[5]This muscle, together with the sternocleidomastoid and the platysma, are important to the dental auxiliary when doing a head and neck examination. See figure on page 33.

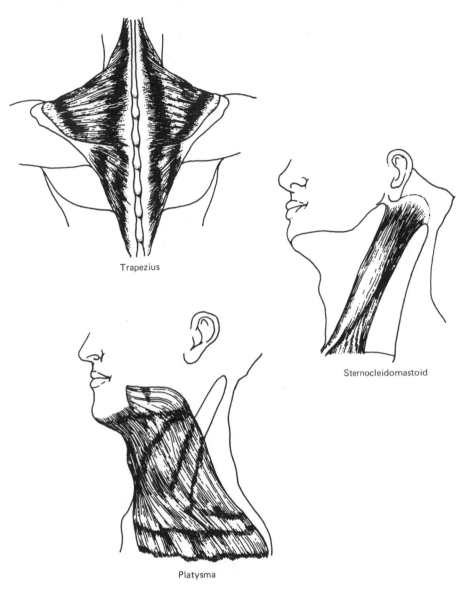

Trapezius

Sternocleidomastoid

Platysma

The trapezius, sternocleidomastoid, and platysma muscles shown are of particular importance to dentistry.

Muscle	Location and Function
Sacrospinalis	The (sa″-crō-spi′-nalis) is a large muscular, tendinous mass on either side of the vertebral column in the thoracic and cervical region beneath the trapezius and the latissimus dorsi muscles.
Serratus anterior	The (ser′-rā-tus) anterior is a thin muscular sheet between the ribs and the scapula. It spreads over the lateral part of

Muscle	*Location and Function*
Serratus anterior (continued)	the chest. It draws the scapula forward and rotates the scapula to raise the shoulder when extending the arm.
External and internal intercostals	These muscles fill the spaces between the ribs. They increase and decrease the volume of the thoracic cavity.
Diaphragm	The diaphragm is a dome-shaped muscle that forms the floor of the thoracic cavity and the roof of the abdominal cavity.
External or descending obliques	These muscles are the strongest and the most superficial of the abdominal muscles. Beneath lie the internal or ascending oblique muscles. These muscles, together with other muscles, form a strong support for the abdominal viscera. They assist in compressing the abdominal contents during delivery of the fetus from the body, and during defecation, micturition, and emesis; they also aid in flexing the thorax and pelvis, in lateral bending, and rotation of the spine.
Biceps	The biceps are long cordlike muscles on the anterior surface of the arms. These muscles raise and draw the humerus forward, flex the elbow, and turn the forearm and hand palm upward.
Triceps	The triceps are situated on the dorsal aspect of the arm. They extend the entire length of the dorsal surface of the humerus. These muscles extend the forearm and flex it toward the midline.
Gluteus maximus	The gluteus maximus is the chief muscle of the buttocks. It assists in maintaining an erect position; it acts as a powerful extensor of the hip joint; and it rotates the femur outward and the thigh inward. These muscles are very important in walking and running.
Adductors	There are four muscles in this group. They are located on the inner thighs. Their functions are to flex and rotate the thighs, bring the thighs toward the median line, and flex the legs.
Sartorius	This muscle is a long ribbonlike muscle on the front of the thigh. It crosses the thigh obliquely, and the function of this muscle is to flex the hip and knee joint. It also rotates the thigh outward.
Quadriceps femoris	This muscle covers the anterior aspect of the thigh. It extends the leg and rotates the thigh outward.
Biceps femoris	These muscles along with the semitendinosus and semimembranosus muscles are known as the "hamstring muscles." They cover the back of the thigh and assist in flexing the leg and extending the thigh.
Gastrocnemius and soleus	The (gas″-trok-nē′-me-us) and soleus muscles together form the major part of the calf of the leg. Their functions are to flex the ankle and knee joint.

Muscle	*Location and Function*
Tibialis anterior	The (tib″-ē-a′-lis) muscle is on the anterior aspect of the leg. It assists in flexing and inverting the foot.

NEW WORDS

Abduction (ab-dukt′-tion): The drawing away from the midline.

Defecation: The voiding of excrement.

Emesis: Vomiting.

Micturition (mik″-tu-rish′-un): The act of urinating.

SELF—TEST

1. Muscular tissue is classified as what kind of tissue? _____

2. Name and define the three characteristics of muscular tissue. _____

_____

3. What are the two movement classifications of muscular tissue? _____

_____

4. Why is muscular tissue classified in the above manner? _____

5. Are most skeletal muscles paired? _____

6. What is meant by *muscle tone*? _____

7. Explain *tetany*. _____

8. What does the glycogen stored in the cells do for muscular tissue? _____

_____

9. What three muscles, in this group of muscles, are important to the dental auxiliary? _____

10. Where are the above muscles located and give at least one function of

each. _____

_____

_____

The Respiratory System

Almost all living things require a continual supply of oxygen. It is a well-known fact that a human being can live a few weeks without food and a few days without water, but only a few minutes without oxygen. Oxygen is fuel for the cells of the body. If deprived of oxygen, the cells of the central nervous system will die in 4 to 6 minutes, most body processes will stop, and death soon follows.

In humans, air is inhaled through the nose or mouth. The air then proceeds down the pharynx, enters the trachea, and then goes on to the lungs. In the lungs the circulating blood comes into contact with the inspired air and takes up oxygen. As this oxygenated blood travels through the body, it gives up the oxygen to the cells and takes up carbon dioxide—the end product of chemical change within the cells—which is ultimately expelled from the nose or the mouth. This action is known as an "exchange of gases" and is called *respiration.*

Where does this vital gas, oxygen, come from? It comes from plant life, both on land and in the sea.

The organs of the respiratory system are described in the list below. The location and function of each are included.

Organs	*Location and Function*
Nose	The nose is not only the organ of smell but is also a passageway for air going to and from the lungs. The external part of the nose is a triangular framework of bone and cartilage covered with skin. On the inferior surface there are two oval-shaped openings called nostrils or nares. Internally the nose is lined with mucous membrane. It is divided into two spaces by the nasal septum, which very often is deviated. On the right and left lateral walls of the nose are the conchae (kong'-kē), which are spongy scroll-like bones that increase the surface over which the air travels and thus allow the air to be warmed by the warm, rich blood supply located just under the surface of the mucous membrane. In the mucus-coated cilia, bacteria and dust are also entrapped and are thus prevented from passing into the lungs.
Pharynx	The (far'-inks) is the posterior passageway from the nose that allows air to travel from the nose to the larynx and on to the lungs. There are three sections to the pharynx: (1) the nasopharynx, upper part, (2) the oropharynx, middle part, and (3) the laryngeal (la-rin'-gē-al) pharynx, lower part. The pharynx is about 5 inches (12.5 cm) long. It is covered with mucous membrane and ciliated epithelium to entrap dust and bacteria.
Larynx	The larynx is the voice box. It lies in the anterior part of the neck in front of the pharynx. It is composed of fibro-cartilage, elastic ligaments, and muscles. The three principal cartilages are the cricoid, thyroid, and the epiglottis. The cricoid, a ringlike cartilage, forms the lower and back part of the larynx. The thyroid is the largest of the three and is composed of two square plates joined to form the laryngeal prominence called the *Adam's apple.* The epiglottis acts as a lid folding down and over the glottis to prevent food from entering the trachea during deglutition. (The glottis is the opening between the vocal cords that allows air to pass into the trachea and on to the lungs.

Organs	Location and Function
Trachea	The trachea is also known as the *windpipe*. It is a fibrous muscular tube about 4 inches (10 cm) long. It lies in front of the esophagus and extends from the larynx downward, where it then divides into two tubes called the *bronchi*. The walls of the trachea are lined with mucous membrane and ciliated epithelium. This epithelium protects the lungs from impurities.
Bronchi	There are two bronchi, one right and one left. The right one is the shortest, widest, and most nearly vertical. The bronchi enter the right or the left lung and then divide into a number of smaller branches called *bronchial tubes* or *bronchioles*. Each bronchiole terminates in an enlargement called the *atrium*. Each atrium is a series of saclike projections known as *alveoli* or *air cells*.
Lungs	The lungs are cone-shaped, porous, spongy organs in the right and left chambers of the thoracic cavity. The heart lies between them. The right lung is larger and heavier and also broader owing to the inclination of the heart to the left side.
Pleura	The (ploo'-rah) is a thin, serous membranous sac that invests the lungs (pulmonary pleura) and lines the walls of the thoracic cavity (parietal pleura). Both layers are moistened by serum to prevent friction during respiration.

Respiration. The purpose of respiration is to supply the cells with oxygen and to rid them of excess carbon dioxide, to equalize the temperature of the body, and to eliminate excess water. About one pint of water is eliminated daily via this system. Breathing is a series of inspirations and expirations. Inspiration is the result of contraction of muscles, and expiration is mainly passive. Unlike the beat of the heart, the contractions of the respiratory muscles are entirely dependent on the nervous system, especially that part known as the *medulla oblongata*. The action of the respiratory system is automatic. When the respiratory center detects an increased amount of carbon dioxide in the blood, the rate and depth of the respirations are increased so that the lungs are ventilated. To some extent, breathing can be controlled by the will. The average respiration rate for an adult is anywhere from 14 to 18 breaths per minute. During the first year the respirations are between 44 and 45, at age 5 they are about 26 per minute, and at age 15 they are about 25. However, exercise can increase the respiratory rate.

External Respiration. External respiration takes place in the lungs; it consists of the passage of oxygen from the alveoli to the blood, and the elimination of carbon dioxide from the blood to the alveoli.

Internal Respiration. Internal respiration takes place in all of the cells that make up the body tissues. It is the passage of oxygen from the blood to the cells, and the elimination of carbon dioxide from the cells to the blood.

NEW WORDS

Tidal air: The amount of air that flows in and out with each respiration.

Apnea (ap'-nē-ah): Temporary stopping of breathing.

Cilia: Hairlike processes found on many cells, capable of a vibratory or lashing movement.

Deglutition (de'-glu-ti-tion): Act of swallowing.

Dyspnea (disp-nē'-ah): Difficult or labored breathing.

Eupnea (up-ne'-ah): Normal respiration.

Hyperpnea (hi'-perp-nē'-ah): Increased depth and rate of respiration.

The drawing below shows the major parts of the respiratory system.

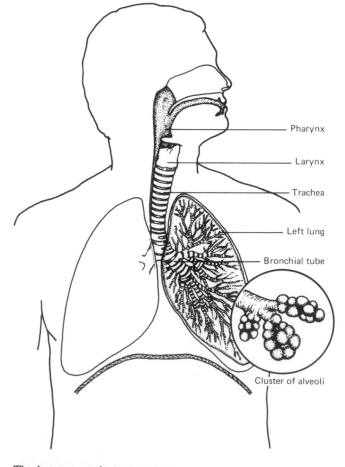

Pharynx

Larynx

Trachea

Left lung

Bronchial tube

Cluster of alveoli

The human respiratory system.

1. Where does the oxygen we breathe come from? _____

2. What are the nares? _____

3. Name the three sections of the pharynx. Locate them. _____
_____

4. Are the nose and the pharynx lined with ciliated epithelium? If so, what is the function of the cilia? _____
_____

5. Which cartilage in the voice box is called the *Adam's apple*? _____

6. What is the technical name for the windpipe? _____

7. Where does the heart lie in the thoracic cavity in relationship to the lungs?
_____

8. What is the pleura? _____

9. What is the purpose of respiration? _____

10. Is the act of respiration always involuntary? Explain. _____
_____

11. How many respirations are average for the infant, child, teenager, adult?
_____

12. Explain the difference between external and internal respiration. _____
_____

13. Define the following: tidal air, apnea, deglutition, eupnea, hyperpnea.
_____
_____
_____
_____

The Digestive System

The human body requires water, carbohydrates, proteins, fats, minerals, and vitamins to survive. These substances must be supplied by the food ingested. They cannot be synthesized in their natural form, and therefore they must be split into simpler substances. This action takes place in the digestive tract. In humans, the digestive tract, or *alimentary canal*, is essentially a tube beginning with the mouth and ending with the anus. This canal is designed as a series of regions with sphincter (control) valves to control the passage of food. Although food when chewed is somewhat broken down, it is not soluble enough to pass through the wall of the digestive tract and on to the individual tissue cells. Therefore, through the aid of accessory organs such as the liver and the pancreas, and with the aid of various chemical and physical actions, the food passes through each region from mouth to anus, with each region doing its part to convert the food into substances the tissue cells can utilize.

The list below describes the major parts of the digestive tract giving the location and function of each.

Digestive Tract	Location and Function
Oral cavity	Digestion begins in the oral cavity. First the food is mixed with saliva from the salivary glands to moisten and lubricate it. The saliva contains the enzyme ptyalin (ti̅′-ah-lin), which partially digests starch by converting it to maltose and dextrose. The tongue then pushes the food back toward the oropharynx, which leads into the esophagus.
Esophagus	The esophagus is a straight hollow tube about 8 inches (20 cm) long. It extends from the lower part of the pharynx to the stomach. It secretes mucus to protect the lining mucosa from abrasive food. Upon reaching the middle third of the esophagus, a series of muscular contractions in the esophagus push the food on to the stomach. This action takes place in about 7 seconds.
Stomach	The stomach is a collapsible, muscular, saclike portion of the digestive tract, located between the esophagus and the small intestine. It is a temporary reservoir for large amounts of food. Lining the mucous membrane of the stomach are gastric glands that secrete gastric fluid—a fluid that contains hydrochloric acid, pepsin, and small amounts of other enzymes needed to convert food into substances that are soluble and readily absorbed by the small intestine. Although digestion continues in the stomach, very little absorption takes place. Alcohol and some condiments appear to be the only substances absorbed by the stomach. A series of wave-like movements, contractions and relaxations, called *peristalsis* (per″-i-stal′-sis), thoroughly mix the gastric juices with the food until it becomes a milky white substance called *chyme* (kime). The chyme is then forwarded on to the next region—the small intestine—where most of the digestion of food takes place.
Small intestine	The so-called small intestine is really a narrow coiled tube about 20 to 23 feet (7 m) long. This is where absorption, or the passage of digested food material from the digestive tract to the blood, takes place. Throughout the whole length of the small intestine there are minute fingerlike projections called *villi*. After food is digested, it passes through the cells on the surface of the villi and into the blood vessels or the lymph vessels where it eventually enters into the main cir-

Digestive Tract	Location and Function
Small intestine (continued)	culating system. Again, by a series of peristalic movements, the portion of the chyme that has not been absorbed is forwarded to the large colon for excretion. Secretions from the liver and the pancreas (accessory organs) also aid in digestion. *Duodenum*: The (du'-o-de'-num) is the first part of the small intestine, leading from the stomach to the second portion of the small intestine. Both the common bile duct and the pancreatic duct empty into it.
Liver	The liver is an accessory organ. One of its digestive functions is the manufacture of bile from the blood. The gallbladder serves as a reservoir for the bile. When stimulated, the stored bile empties via the duodenum into the small intestine, and the bile salts begin their emulsifying action on the fats.
Pancreas	The pancreas is an accessory digestive organ also. It lies below and behind the stomach and the liver. The secretions of the pancreas contain large amounts of amylase for digesting carbohydrates, trypsinogen for digesting proteins, and lipase for digesting fats. In addition to the digestive enzymes, pancreatic secretions contain large amounts of sodium bicarbonate, which reacts with the hydrochloric acid from the stomach to form sodium chloride and carbonic acid. The carbonic acid is absorbed into the blood and becomes water and carbon dioxide. The carbon dioxide is expired through the lungs.[6] A special group of cells in the pancreas, called the *islands of Langerhans*, secrete the hormone insulin, which aids in carbohydrate metabolism.
Large intestine	The large intestine is only about 5 feet (1.5 m) long, but it is wider than the small intestine. The principal function of the large intestine is to collect and dispose of materials not digested. Previously undigested food is passed from the small intestine to the large by peristalsis, then on to the colon and the rectum, where it is eliminated through the external opening called the *anus*. Most of the water has been absorbed in the large intestine, and the material excreted is mostly solids. This material is called *feces*.

[6]Arthur C. Guyton, *Function of the Human Body*, 2nd ed. (Philadelphia: W. B. Saunders Company, 1965), p. 330.

The illustration below locates the major parts of the human digestive system.

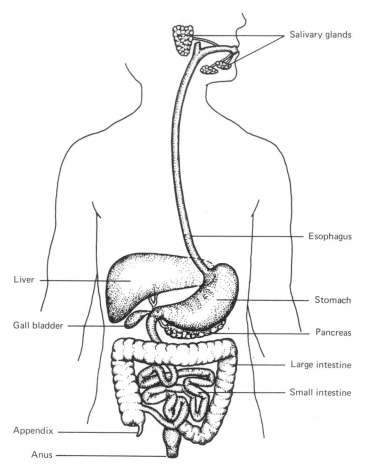

The human digestive system.

SELF—TEST

1. Name six substances man must ingest to survive. _____

_____

2. Where does digestion begin? _____

3. What enzyme does saliva contain? _____

4. What is the term for the wavelike contractions that propel food from the esophagus to the anus? _____

5. Where does most digestion take place? _____

6. Give the definition and function of the villi, and tell where they are found. _____

_____

7. What is one function of the liver? _____

8. What is one function of the pancreas? _____

9. What is the principal function of the large intestine? _____

10. What are feces? _____

11. Where is the hormone insulin found, and what is its function? _____

_____

12. Where is the duodenum located? _____

13. What is the function of the gallbladder? _____

The Excretory System: Urinary Tract

The excretory system actually involves many excretory organs—including the lungs that excrete carbon dioxide and some water, the alimentary canal that excretes solid wastes, the skin that excretes water and salt, and the kidneys that excrete water and waste products in the form of urine. However, in this section only the urinary system will be discussed. The list below describes the major parts of the urinary tract giving the location and functions of each.

Urinary Tract	Location and Function
Kidneys	The kidneys are two bean-shaped glandular organs at the back of the abdominal cavity at approximately waist level. There is one on each side of the spinal column. The kidneys are embedded in fatty tissue, which is one of their chief supporting structures. Near the concave center of these bean-shaped organs is a fissure that is called the *hilum*. This fissure allows the ureter to enter the kidneys, and it provides an entrance and exit for the blood vessels, lymph vessels, and nerves. The kidneys' chief functions are to maintain normal composition of the blood and to remove waste in the form of urine.
Nephrons	In each kidney are approximately one million nephrons (intricately coiled tubes). These tubes are the basic functional units of the kidney. Their function is to remove certain waste products from the blood plasma, and to allow for re-absorption of water and some electrolytes back into the blood, thus assisting in the maintenance of normal fluid balance in the body. The water and the solutes that remain form urine.
Ureters	The (ū-rē′-ters) are two narrow muscular tubes that conduct urine by peristalic movement from the kidneys to the urinary bladder.

Urinary Tract	Location and Function
Urinary bladder	This is a hollow muscular organ situated in the pelvic cavity. It is a reservoir for the reception of urine. It holds about 200 to 400 ml.
Urethra	The (ū-rē'-thra) is the canal that extends from the bladder to the outside of the body. It differs in length and function in the male and female. In the female it is a very short membranous canal about 1½ inches (3.5 cm) long. It is located just superior to the vagina for the purpose of conveying urine from the bladder to the exterior of the body. In the male it is about 7½ inches (19 cm) long and extends down the penis. It has a combined function in the male: the conveying of spermatozoa and the emptying of the bladder.

Urine. Urine, the end product of the urinary system, is about 95% water. Normally, it is a transparent yellowish liquid that contains water and waste. However, diet and/or disease may change the color and create a cloudy appearance.

NEW WORDS

Solute (sol'-ūt): A substance that is dissolved in a liquid to form a solution.

Electrolytes: Any compound that, when dissolved in water, separates into changed particles capable of conducting an electrical current. They play an essential role in the working of a cell, maintaining fluid and normal acid base balance. Sodium is one example. It is a key regulator in water balance and in the normal functioning of muscles and nerves.

The illustration on page 45 shows the location of the major parts of the human urinary system.

SELF—TEST

1. Where are the kidneys located? _____

2. What is the chief function of the kidneys? _____

_____

3. Where are the nephrons, and what is their function? _____

_____

4. What are ureters, and what is their function? _____

_____

5. Where is the urinary bladder located? _____

6. Give the location and function(s) of the urethra in the female and the male. _____

_____

7. Normally what is the color of urine? _____

8. Define *solute*. _____

9. Give one example of an electrolyte that is a key regulator in water balance and normal functioning of muscles and nerves. _____

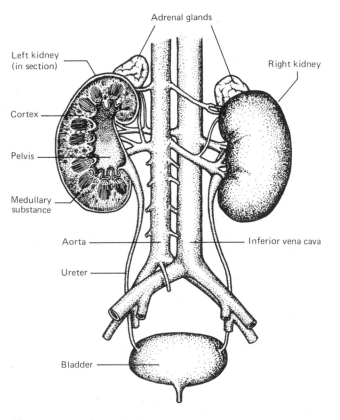

The human urinary system.

The Circulatory Systems

In order to survive, the human body must take in nutrients, process them, and then eliminate the wastes. These functions are handled very well by the digestive and urinary systems. The body must also breathe in oxygen and exhale carbon dioxide. The respiratory system takes very good care of this function. One function not provided by the above systems is the transportation of the nutrients and water and oxygen from the external environment to the internal, and vice versa. This is the function of the circulatory systems.

The human body, as you can see, is a community with all systems working together to keep this fantastic machine functioning.

The General Circulatory System. The *heart* is the center of the general circulatory system; its function is to pump the blood which is carrying the substances needed by the cells, through a closed system of vessels to all parts of the body. The heart lies behind the sternum (breast bone) and slightly to the left. It is a hollow, muscular organ about the size of a fist. It is a tireless organ beating approximately 72 times per minute, or about 100,000 times per day, year in and year out with only a few seconds rest between each beat. This hollow muscular organ has three layers of tissue lining its walls. The outermost layer is the *pericardium* (peri'-kär'-di-um); the inner layer is the *endocardium* (en'-do-kär'-di-um); and the third layer is the muscle of the heart itself. This layer is called the *myocardium* (my'-o-kär'-di-um). The heart is divided into four chambers. There are two small upper chambers called the *atria*, and two lower chambers called the *ventricles*. The right atrium and right ventricle are separated from the left atrium and left ventricle by a wall of muscle called a *septum*. Actually the heart is a double pump with the right side handling the venous blood and the left side the arterial blood. There are four very important valves, two of which are located, one on each side of the heart, between the atrium and the ventricle; two more are located, one each at the entrances to the aorta and to the pulmonary artery. These one-way valves are there to regulate the direction in which the blood flows. Thus, normally, blood can flow only from the veins to the atria, from the atria to the ventricles, and from the ventricles to the arteries.

To trace the route that blood takes, as it circulates, begin with the dark red venous blood, or used blood, which has been returned to the heart via the large vein immediately above the heart called the *superior vena cava*. This vein drains the blood from the head and arms, while the *inferior vena cava*, immediately below the heart, drains the blood from the lower parts of the body. The two vena cavae then drain into the right atrium. From the right atrium the blood is forced into the right ventricle, which contracts and forces the venous blood up and into the right and left branches of the pulmonary artery and then on to both lungs where it exchanges, for oxygen, the carbon dioxide that was picked up from the body's tissues. This fresh oxygen changes the color of the blood from dark red to bright red. It is then called *oxygenated blood*. This oxygenated blood is returned to the heart via the right and left pulmonary veins, which drain into the left atrium. From there the blood drains into the left ventricle, which contracts, forcing this fresh blood into the aorta and on through the arterioles and the capillaries, carrying fresh blood to each cell in the body and collecting wastes for the return trip to the lungs via the venules. The *venules* are small vessels that receive blood from the capillary plexus and then join to form veins. These veins ultimately empty into the superior and inferior vena cavae. The blood used by the heart takes a different route: it drains through the coronary sinus, which is the terminal portion of the great cardiac vein, and then into the lungs. Blood entering the heart goes via the coronary arteries, which are the first branches of the aorta. The illustration on page 47 locates the major parts of the human heart.

The Portal Circulatory System. By a complex route, venous blood from the digestive organs, the spleen, and the pancreas is detoured, and for a very good

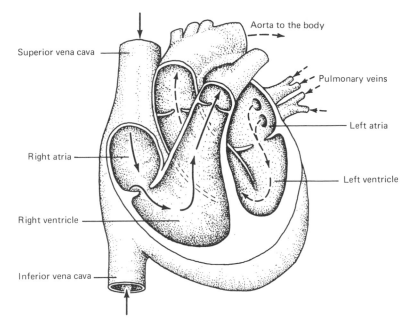

Aorta to the body

Superior vena cava

Pulmonary veins

Left atria

Right atria

Left ventricle

Right ventricle

Inferior vena cava

The human heart, showing the route blood will take.

reason. Billions of bacteria enter the blood from the gastrointestinal tract and must be eliminated. So venous blood is sent via the portal vein into the liver for cleansing. The nutritive blood that the liver uses enters the liver by way of the hepatic artery, so that nutrients may be altered and in some cases stored. "Normally the liver cells remove approximately 2/3 of the glucose that has been absorbed into the portal blood from the intestines and perhaps as much as 1/2 of the proteins . . . ."[7] These nutrients are reserved for future use. This small amount of simple protein, according to Dr. Guyton, should probably be referred to as amino acids since current information indicates that amino acids are stored, to some extent, as simple protein.[8]

All of this conditioned blood leaves the liver via the hepatic vein, drains into the inferior vena cava, and then enters the main circulatory system.

Blood. Blood is the red, sticky liquid vehicle that carries nourishment and oxygen to all parts of the body and carries away waste. It is the medium for the interchange of gases; it transmits internal secretions that control the chemical activities of cells; it equalizes the temperature and the water content of the body; and it aids in protecting the body from toxic substances. The quantity in the human body is determined by the size and weight of the individual. An average adult will have from 5 to 6 quarts of blood. The fluid

[7]Arthur C. Guyton, *Function of the Human Body*, 2nd ed. (Philadelphia: W.B. Saunders Company, 1965), p. 148.

[8]Ibid.

medium of blood is called *plasma*. Suspended in the plasma are formed elements, which include cells, or corpuscles, and platelets.

Formed Elements. Blood consists of a fluid medium called *plasma*, in which minute structures called *formed elements* are suspended. A description of these elements follows:

Red Blood Cells. Red blood cells are called *erythrocytes*. During maturation the nucleus of the erythrocyte is eliminated. It is then known as a *corpuscle* (kor'-pus-l). Without a nucleus, red corpuscles cannot reproduce. Young red cells called *erythroblasts*, however, do have nuclei and do reproduce, but they are not found in the circulating blood. After birth, erythrocytes (RBC) form in the bone marrow; then when they lose their nuclei, they pass into the circulating system. Every second, millions of new red blood cells pass from the bone marrow into the bloodstream, while other millions of cells are removed in the liver and the spleen. The red blood corpuscles are the carriers of oxygen to the body tissues, a function that depends on the hemoglobin present in the erythrocytes. These same cells transport carbon dioxide from the body tissues to be eliminated via the lungs.

White Blood Cells. White blood cells (WBC) are called *leukocytes*. There are several types of leukocytes. In general their function is to protect the body from pathogenic bacteria. They also appear to play a role in promoting tissue repair. These cells are mainly produced in the bone marrow, lymph nodes, and the spleen. Almost as many leukocytes are produced as erythrocytes in the bone marrow. However, there are far fewer in circulation. This is because they exist only for a very short time, since as they perform their function of protecting the body through the process of phagocytosis, they are destroyed.

Platelets. Platelets are also called *thrombocytes*. They are small platelike structures, from which threads of fibrin, an insoluble protein, radiate. They are much smaller than the erythrocytes and the leukocytes, and, because fibrin is essential to the clotting of blood these small platelets play a key role.

Plasma. After the erythrocytes, leukocytes, and platelets are removed from the blood, there remains a transparent, slightly viscous, amber liquid called *plasma*. This liquid contains proteins, carbohydrates, fats, and mineral salts. One of the very important proteins in plasma is fibrinogen, which produces fibrin in response to substances released from the platelets. When there is an injury that causes blood loss, fibrin, a tangled network of minute threads, shrinks to form a hard clot. This clotting reaction is very necessary to preserve life; but for some persons called *bleeders* (hemophiliacs), clotting is much slower because the necessary factors for the coagulation of blood are not present. Therefore these people can bleed to death. This is a hereditary disease.

The clotting reaction can also be dangerous. If a clot should form within a blood vessel (thrombus) and block the blood supply to a vital organ, a condition known as *thrombosis* would occur. If a clot or a fragment of a clot (embolus) should break loose and enter the bloodstream, blocking a blood vessel, a condition known as an *embolism* would occur. Either of these conditions can be life-threatening.

Serum. Serum is the clear liquid that separates from the blood when it is allowed to clot. It is plasma from which fibrinogen has been removed during the process of clotting. This occurs when the clot has formed and the fibrin threads contract, expressing plasma out of the clot. So, essentially, serum is the clear portion of plasma after the solid elements have been removed. Serum remains fluid.

Tissue Fluid. Tissue fluid is a liquid substance that surrounds the cells. It is low in protein. It is formed by filtration through the capillaries, and it drains away as lymph.

Blood Pressure. Blood pressure is the pressure of the blood on the walls of the arteries. When the ventricles contract, a shock wave travels along the arteries. This is the pulse that one feels. Normally blood pressure is constant. However, fright, exercising vigorously, or experiencing nervous tension will all increase the pressure of the blood on arterial walls. The body has one well-known regulating device for meeting stress, and that is adrenaline (ad-ren'-ah-lin), a hormone that is released into the blood by the adrenal glands. These glands and their action will be discussed later.

Arteries. There are many arteries, arterioles, and capillaries. Only a few will be discussed here. Those supplying the face, neck, and dental apparatus will be discussed in more detail in Chapter 2.

Listed below are the arteries where a pulse can be felt, or where hemorrhaging can be stopped by applying pressure.

Artery	Location
Radial	On the thumb side of the wrist.
Facial	Where the facial artery passes over the jawbone.
Temporal	Above and to the outer side of the outer canthus of the eye.
Common carotid	On either side of the neck along the front edge of the sternocleidomastoid muscle.
Brachial	On the inner margin of the biceps muscle at the bend of the elbow.
Femoral	In the upper three-fourths of the thigh where the femoral artery crosses the brim of the pelvis.
Dorsalis pedia	At the dorsum of the foot just below the ankle joint.

Aorta. The aorta is the great artery arising from the left ventricle. It is the main trunk of the arterial system. It arches over the root of the left lung and descends along the vertebral column, then passes through the abdominal cavity, and finally divides into the right and left iliac arteries. There are many branches along the way.

Veins. Like the arteries, there are many veins and venules (small veins), but only a few will be discussed. The veins are designed, as previously stated, to carry blood to the heart; therefore they are sometimes used to carry materials quickly into the bloodstream by intravenous injection, or they can be used to remove blood for examination. There are three veins, as defined below, that the dental auxiliary should be aware of as they are the ones most frequently used for these purposes.

Median Cubital. The median cubital lies below the elbow. It passes obliquely upward across the cubital fossa.
Cephalic. The cephalic begins in the dorsal venous network on the dorsum of the hand and ascends the radial side of the forearm.
Basilic. The basilic begins in the dorsal network on the dorsum of the hand and extends upward along the posterior part of the ulnar side of the forearm, ending a little above the elbow.

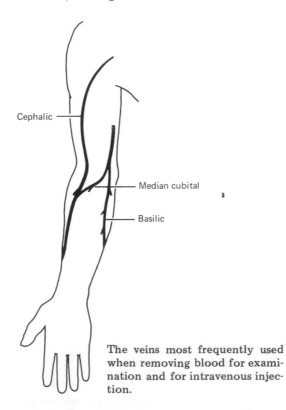

Cephalic

Median cubital

Basilic

The veins most frequently used when removing blood for examination and for intravenous injection.

The Lymphatic System. Tissue fluid bathing the cells and waste products from the cells must both be removed, filtered, and returned to the blood circulatory system. This is the function of the lymphatic capillaries, the lymphatic vessels, and the lymph nodes, which are scattered throughout the body. The lymph capillaries lie in the tissue fluid, in the intercellular spaces, where they collect excess fluid, waste products, and other debris, and then transport these in the form of *lymph*, a clear fluid, through an intricate system of lymphatic vessels and strategically placed filtering stations called *lymph nodes*, to finally empty into the subclavian veins and the blood circulatory system. As the lymph passes through the lymph nodes (small grouped masses of lymphoid tissue containing many lymphocytes), the lymph is filtered, and pathogenic organisms, malignant cells, and dead blood cells normally are removed.

Sometimes included in this system are the so-called lymphatic organs: the spleen, the tonsils, and the thymus—the reason being that these organs are composed of large masses of lymphoid tissue, and they appear to perform some of the same functions as the lymphatic system.

Spleen. The spleen is a highly vascular organ that acts as a reservoir for red blood cells; in times of need, it releases the red blood cells into the bloodstream. It lies beneath the diaphragm, behind and to the left of the stomach. It contains lymphoid tissue. It is thought to destroy used-up red blood corpuscles and to preserve the iron released from them. It also serves as a filtering station.

Tonsils. The tonsils are masses of lymphoid tissue situated in the throat and nasopharynx. They act as filtering stations.

Thymus. The thymus is included here because of its large mass of lymphoid tissue and because of the large numbers of lymphocytes present. It consists of two lobes that lie partly in the neck and partly in the thorax. It appears to play a role in immunity and it does manufacture lymphocytes.

SELF—TEST

1. What is the main organ of the circulatory system? _____

2. Where is this main organ located? _____

3. Name the three layers of tissue lining the walls of the heart. _____

_____

4. Which side of the heart handles the venous blood? The arterial blood?

_____

5. What color is venous blood? Arterial blood? Why? _____

6. Why is venous blood routed through the liver? _____

7. How much blood does the average adult have? What influences this amount? _____

_____

8. What are erythrocytes? Where do they form? _____

9. What is the function of the RBC? _____

10. What are the WBC called? What is their primary function? _____

11. Give another name for platelets. What is their key role? _____

12. What is meant by *hemophiliac*? _____

13. What is a thrombus? _____

14. What is an embolus? _____

15. Define *blood pressure*. _____

16. Tell where the following arteries are located: radial, facial, temporal, common carotid, brachial, femoral, dorsalis pedia. _____

_____

_____

_____

17. What is the name of the great artery? _____

18. Name the three veins that are most frequently used for intravenous injections (IVs) or for blood samples. _____

_____

19. What is the function of the lymph capillaries and the nodes? _____

_____

20. What organs are associated with the lymphatic system? _____

The Endocrine System

The endocrine system is a system of ductless glands that effects control over certain bodily functions by releasing secretions called *hormones*. These hormones are then carried to the organ or cells that require a specific hormone in order to function.

Some other hormones released by organs—hormones that do not belong to this system—include insulin from the pancreas, estrogen and progesterone from the ovaries, and testosterone from the testes. These were discussed earlier. The following list defines glands of the endocrine system.

Gland	Location and Function
Thyroid	The thyroid is a small, flat gland near the forepart of the trachea. This gland produces thyroxin from small amounts of iodine. However, there generally is not enough iodine in the water we consume, so to be certain we ingest the iodine needed to produce thyroxin, iodized salt can be used. An insufficiency could result in goiter. The thyroid hormone also affects the utilization of fats by the body, and increases or decreases the metabolic rate depending on how much thyroxin is released into the blood. It affects the heart by increasing its metabolism. It also affects the nervous system by increasing the rate of activity, which can cause muscle

Gland	*Location and Function*
Thyroid (continued)	tremor. The gastrointestinal tract is also affected, resulting in diarrhea or constipation.
Parathyroids	There are four parathyroids. These are small red-brown bodies near the thyroid gland that regulate calcium metabolism. The hormone secreted is called *parathormone*. One of its functions is to control the depositon of and the retention of calcium in the bones. An insufficiency of parathormone can cause mental or cardiac disturbances.
Adrenal	The adrenal glands are two in number, one above each kidney. Each gland consists of two parts: (1) the *medulla*, which is part of the sympathetic nervous system and secretes epinephrine (adrenalin) and norephrine; and (2) the *cortex*, which secretes adrenocortical hormones that (a) control electrolyte balances of sodium, chloride, and potassium, (b) affect metabolism of protein, fat, and glucose, and (c) cause masculinizing effects. These glands also prepare the body for energetic action by releasing extra sugar for quick energy in the case of fear. When this occurs, the arteries contract, blood pressure rises, heartbeat and breathing are speeded up, blood clots more quickly, and more oxygen is consumed.
Pituitary	The pituitary gland is known as the *master gland* of the endocrine system. It is about the size of a pea and is located at the base of the brain. It is also called the *hypophysis*. It is connected to the hypothalamus, which controls many of its secretory functions. Many different hormones are produced by this gland, some of which act upon other endocrine glands to stimulte their particular hormones. Some of the other functions of this gland are: growth control, weight control, urine formation control, and muscular control such as contraction of the uterus during labor, and ejection of milk from the mammary glands.

NEW WORDS

Norepinephrine (nor″-ep-i-nef′-rin): A hormone secreted by the adrenal medulla in response to splanchnic stimulation. It is also formed at the endings of certain nerve fibers of the sympathetic nervous system and it takes part in the transmission of impulses from one nerve ending to another.

Splanchnic (sp-langk′-nik): Pertaining to the viscera.

Electrolyte (e-lek′-tro-līt): Any compound that when dissolved in water, separates into charged particles (ions) capable of conducting an electric current. The chief electrolytes in the body are sodium, potassium, and calcium.

The major glands of the human endocrine system are shown on the illustration below. The three glands that have similar functions but are not part of the system are also shown. These glands are the pancreas, ovary and testis.

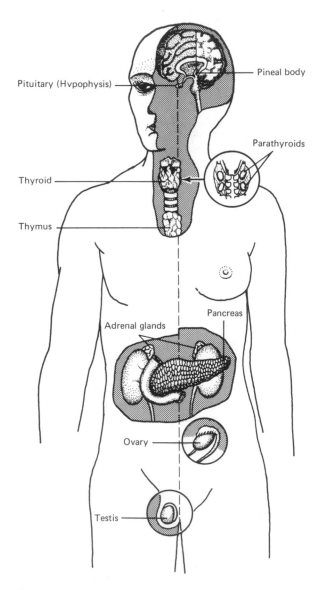

The human endocrine system.

1. What is the name given to the secretions released by the endocrine glands?

2. Name the four major glands of the endocrine system and the three glands that have similar functions but are not part of the system. _____

3. Name the secretions of each major gland, and give its function or functions. _____

4. Which gland is important in dentistry because it regulates calcium metabolism? _____

5. Which gland is known as the master gland? _____

6. Why are glands of the endocrine system known as "ductless" glands?

7. Why is it necessary that there is a sufficiency of iodine in the human diet?

8. Is there generally enough iodine naturally in the food and water we drink?

9. What disease would result in an insufficiency of iodine? _____

10. How can one obtain enough iodine? _____

2

Head and and Neck Anatomy

EMBRYOLOGY OF THE HEAD AND NECK

In Chapter 1 you learned that the entire human body develops from one or more of the three embryonic layers of the blastoderm, and that shortly after conception the embryo is not more than a tube within a tube. As time goes on, however, through proliferation and differentiation of the cells in the three primary layers, a total human being evolves, with structural differentiation being given some precedence over functional differentiation. Rapid growth continues, with the embryo developing from a mere $1/8$ inch (3 mm) at 3 weeks to approximately 4 inches (108 mm) at 16 weeks.

Once the entire neural tube is established, development of the embryo is rapid, with the more noticeable growth lengthwise resulting in the cephalic and caudal ends bending ventrally. The head, or cephalic end, is the first to show further signs of development, with the primitive mouth (stomodeum) occurring about the third week, when the ventral side of the neural tube invaginates and the ectoderm approaches the entoderm with only the buccopharyngeal membrane separating them. (See diagram on page 57.) Soon the buccopharyngeal membrane ruptures, joining the primitive mouth with the primitive digestive tract. Development from here on is so rapid that at two months the embryo is recognizable as a human being.

Branchial Arches

Further development of the embryo results in the appearance of a series of paired lateral outgrowths called branchial arches (resembling gills). There

56

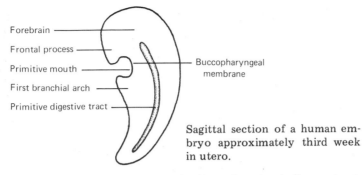

Forebrain
Frontal process
Primitive mouth
First branchial arch
Primitive digestive tract
Buccopharyngeal membrane

Sagittal section of a human embryo approximately third week in utero.

are five of these arches but only four give rise to important structures in the head and neck and only three are of importance to the dental auxiliary as these three are responsible for the further development of various structures in the head and neck. These three are listed below.

Arch I is responsible for the lower lip, mandibular process, muscles of mastication, and the anterior of the tongue.

Arch II is responsible for the side and front of the neck, the posterior part of the tongue, and other associated structures.

Arch III is also responsible for the posterior part of the tongue and other associated structures.

Development of the Face

The development of the face follows an orderly sequence as seen in the illustration below.

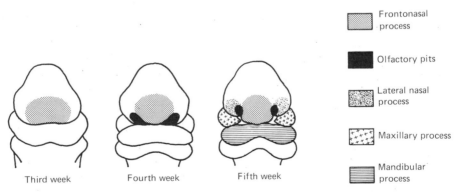

Frontonasal process

Olfactory pits

Lateral nasal process

Maxillary process

Mandibular process

Third week   Fourth week   Fifth week

Frontonasal Process. The frontonasal process appears shortly after the buccopharyngeal membrane ruptures. This prominence appears on the lower anterior portion of the forebrain.

Olfactory Pits. The olfactory pits are formed by deep invaginations on the lower lateral borders of the frontonasal process. They are the future sites of the openings into the nose. They also divide the lower part of the frontonasal process into three parts: the median nasal process and two lateral nasal processes.

Lateral Nasal Processes and Median Nasal Process. The lateral nasal processes become the right and left sides of the nose. The median nasal process becomes the center and tip of the nose. Later on, ingrowth forms the nasal septum. The rounded lateral angles eventually form the globular process.

Globular Process. The globular process occurs through the elongation of the median nasal process. It is a single structure that eventually forms the center of the upper lip (philtrum) and the premaxilla.

Maxillary Process. The maxillary process is formed by a triangular budding at either side of the first branchial arch; also called the *mandibular arch*. This process will eventually form the upper part of the cheeks, lateral part of the upper lip, and part of the nasal cavity; it will also fuse with the nasal processes to form the primitive palate.

Mandibular Process. The mandibular process is formed from the remaining portion of the first branchial arch. It will become the lower part of the cheeks, the mandible, muscles of mastication, and the anterior two-thirds of the tongue. The above processes are located on the figure below.

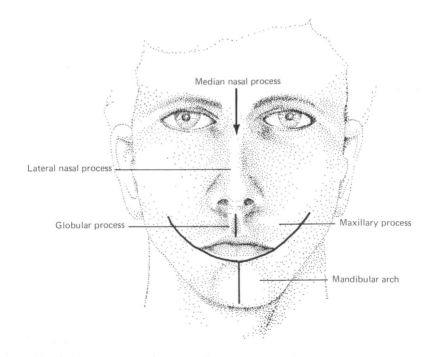

Adult face after the various processes have formed.

NEW WORDS

Branchial (brang′-ke-al): Pertaining to, or resembling, gills.

Stomodeum (sto″-mo-de′-um): The ectodermal depression at the head end of the embryo, which becomes the front part of the mouth.

Invagination: To have one portion (of a hollow organ) drawn back within another.

THE BONES OF THE SKULL

An extensive background in osteology, or the study of bones, is not important to the dental auxiliary. It is important, however, that the student develop a mental picture of how the bones of the skull form the framework for the soft tissues of the cranium, face, and neck.

The skull is composed, essentially, of two classifications of bones: (1) the cranial bones, and (2) the facial bones. There are 8 cranial bones and 14 facial bones, making a total of 22 bones altogether, in the skull.

Cranial Bones

The cranial bones will be discussed first. Numbers of bones are shown in parentheses after each entry.

Bone	Location and Description
Frontal (1) (frun′-tal)	The frontal bone forms the framework for the forehead, the roof between the eyeballs, and the frontal parts of the cerebrum. This bone contains two air spaces called the *frontal sinus.*
Parietal (2) (pah-rī′-e-tal)	The parietal bones form the larger part of the upper and side walls of the cranium (crown of the head).
Temporal (2) (tem′-po-ral)	The temporal bones form the lower sides and part of the base of the central areas of the skull. They also contain the mastoid sinuses and the middle and inner ear.
Ethmoid (1) (eth′-moid)	The ethmoid bone is a delicate, spongy bone. It is located between the eyes, forming a part of the cranial floor and the upper nasal cavities. The superior and middle conchae (kong′-ke) are a part of this bone. They are located on the right and lateral walls of the nasal cavity. This bone contains the two ethmoid sinuses.
Sphenoid (1) (sfe′-noid)	The sphenoid bone is a bat-shaped bone. It is located behind the eyes and forms part of the base of the skull in this region. It extends along the right and left lateral walls, separating the frontal bone from the temporal bones. The lateral wings extend upward to meet with the temporal,

Bone	Location and Description
Sphenoid (continued)	parietal, and frontal bones. These extensions are called the *greater wings of the sphenoid*. This bone contains the two sphenoid sinuses.
Occipital (1) (ok-sip'-ital)	The occipital bone is located at the base of the skull, and it includes most of the base. It is a cuplike bone. Inferiorly and on the midline of this bone there is a large opening called the *foramen magnum*, through which the large nerves and blood vessels pass from the vertebral canal to the cranial cavity. This bone extends at the base to meet with the sphenoid medially, the temporals anteriorly, and the parietal superiorly. The occipital bone also connects with the axis (second cervical vertebra) by strong ligaments.

Study the names of the eight cranial bones as shown on the figure below and then take the Self-Test on the page that follows.

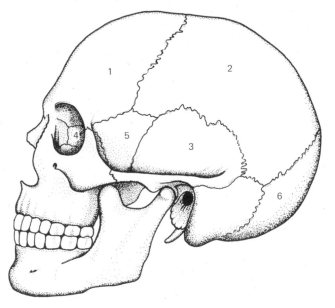

The eight cranial bones. (1) Frontal [1]; (2) parietal [2]; (3) temporal [2]; (4) ethmoid [1]; (5) greater wing of the sphenoid [1]; (6) occipital [1].

Write in the names of the cranial bones on the lines provided below.

1. _____

2. _____

3. _____

4. _____

5. _____

6. _____

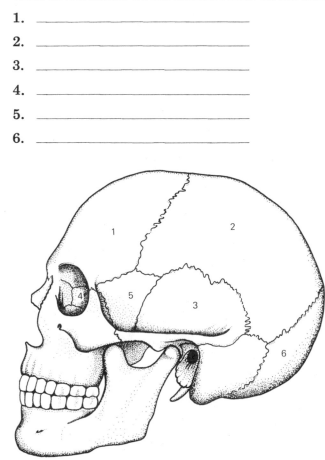

Study the names of the eight individual cranial bones as illustrated, then take the Self-Test on the page that follows.

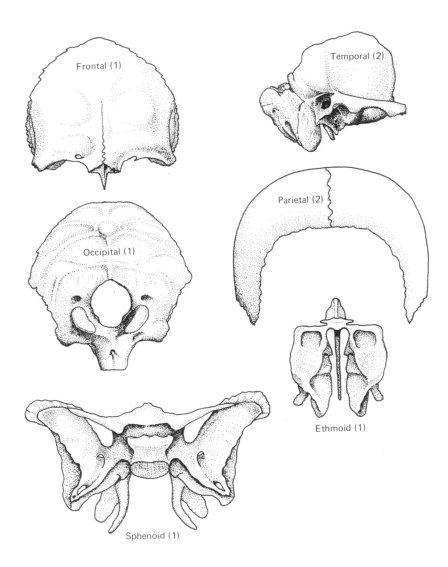

The eight cranial bones. Bones are displayed individually with numbers of parts indicated in parentheses.

On the appropriate illustration write the name and note the number of each individual bone in parentheses.

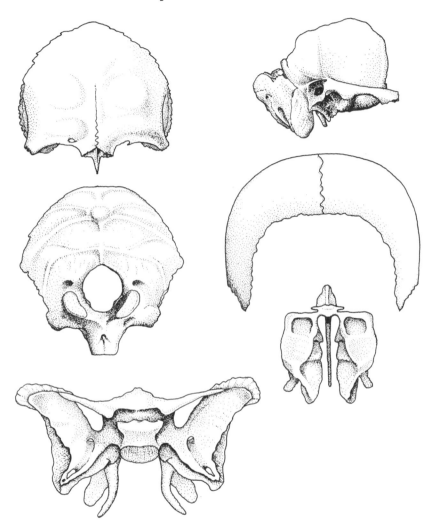

Facial Bones

The following definitions describe the location of each of the fourteen facial bones. Number of bones are inserted in parentheses after entries.

Bone	Location and Description
Maxillae (2) (mak-sil′-e)	The maxillae form the upper jaw. Each maxilla contains rather a large air space called the *maxillary sinus* or the *antrum of Highmore*.

Malar (2) (mā-lar)	The malar bones, or *zygomatic* (zī'-go-mat-ik) *bones* as they are sometimes called, form the higher portion of each cheek. They are also known as the *cheek bones*.
Lacrimal (2) (lak'-ri-mal)	These small bones are found at the inner corner of each orbit. They contain the lacrimal sac and the lacrimal duct (tear duct).
Vomer (1) (vo'-mer)	The vomer forms the inferior and posterior part of the nasal septum.
Palatine (2) (pal'-ah-tīn)	The palatine bones are small L-shaped bones that form the most posterior part of the hard palate and part of the nasal cavity.
Nasal (2) (na'-zal)	The nasal bones form the upper part, or the bridge, of the nose.
Inferior nasal conchae (2)	The inferior nasal conchae are the lowest of the three scroll-like bones that are located on both the right and left lateral walls of the nasal cavity. These bones are also known as *turbinates*. Their purpose is to condition incoming air before it reaches the lungs.
Mandible (1) (man'-di-bl)	The mandible forms the lower jaw. It is the only movable bone in the skull.

Study the names of the 14 facial bones, as shown on the figure, and then take the Self-Test on the following page.

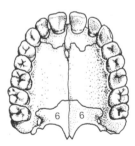

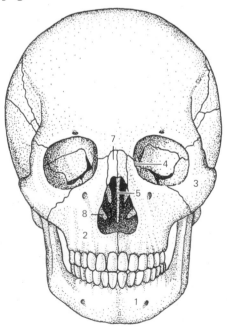

The fourteen facial bones (overall view). (1) Mandible [1]; (2) maxillae [2]; (3) malar (zygomatic [2]; (4) lacrimal [2]; (5) vomer [1]; (6) palatine [2]; (7) nasal [2]; (8) inferior nasal conchae [2].

Write in the names of the various facial bones on the lines provided below.

1. _____

2. _____

3. _____

4. _____

5. _____

6. _____

7. _____

8. _____

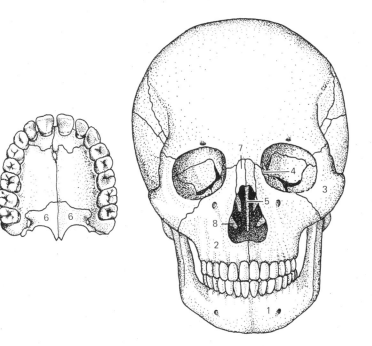

Study the names of the individual facial bones, and then take the Self-Test on the following page.

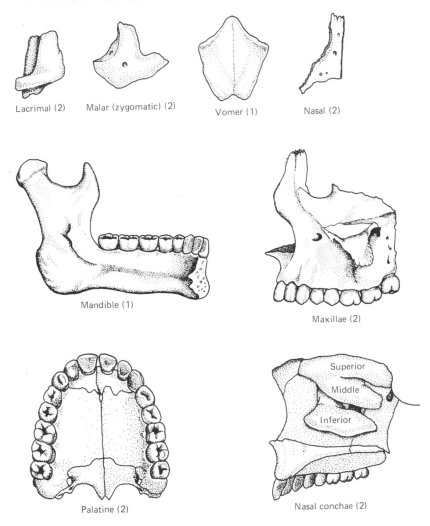

Lacrimal (2)   Malar (zygomatic) (2)   Vomer (1)   Nasal (2)

Mandible (1)

Maxillae (2)

Palatine (2)

Superior
Middle
Inferior

Nasal conchae (2)

The fourteen facial bones. Bones are displayed individually, with numbers of parts indicated in parentheses after each label.

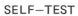

SELF—TEST

Write in the names of each of the individual facial bones on the lines provided in the following diagrams.

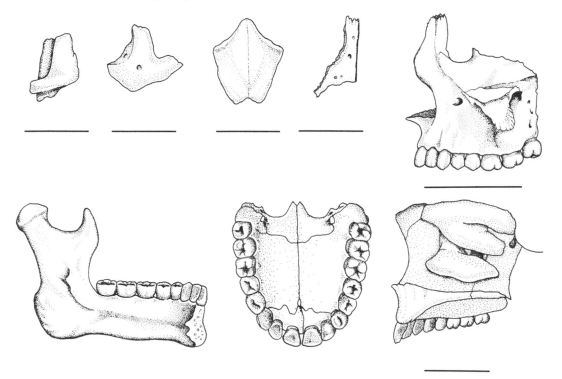

Supplemental Structures of Dental Importance—Frontal View

Name	Location and Description
Supraorbital margins	The ridges just superior to the orbital cavities.
Supraorbital notch (foramen)	A notch at the medial one-third of the supraorbital margin for the supraorbital nerve.
Infraorbital margins	The ridges just inferior to the orbital cavities.
Orbital surfaces of the sphenoid	Surfaces that form the posterior part of the lateral walls of the orbits.
Orbital cavities	The two conical cavities on the anterior surface of the skull that contain the eye, the optic nerve, the muscles of the eyeball, and the lacrimal apparatus.
Canine fossae (fos'-ae)	Depressions on the anterior surface of the mixillae just posterior to the roots of the canine eminences.
Zygomatic foramina (fo-ram'-i-na)	Small foramina on the malar (zygomatic) bones.

Name	Location and Description
Symphysis (sim'-fi-sis)	A faint ridge at the midline of the mandible that indicates the line of junction of the two sections.
Mental protuberance	This structure, inferior to the symphysis and at the midline, is a triangular eminence that is depressed in the center.
Mental tubercle	The raised portion on either side of the depressed area of the mental protuberance.
Coronal suture	The interlocking line that occurs between the frontal and the perietal bones.

NEW WORDS

Eminence: A high place; an elevation.

Foramen (fo-rā'-men): A small opening in bone through which nerves and blood vessels pass.

Tubercle (tu'-ber-k'l): A small knoblike prominence.

Study the names of the supplemental structures of the skull as shown on the following figures and then take the Self-Test that follows.

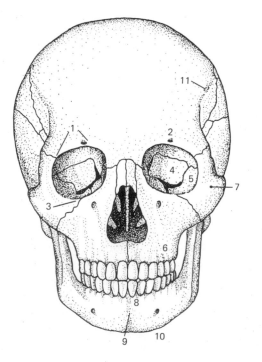

Supplemental structures of dental importance (frontal view). (1) Supraorbital margins; (2) supraorbital notch (foramen); (3) infraorbital margins; (4) orbital surfaces of the sphenoid; (5) orbital cavities; (6) canine fossae; (7) zygomatic foramina; (8) symphysis; (9) mental protuberance; (10) mental tubercle; (11) coronal suture.

Write in the names of the supplemental structures on the lines provided.

1. _____

2. _____

3. _____

4. _____

5. _____

6. _____

7. _____

8. _____

9. _____

10. _____

11. _____

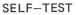

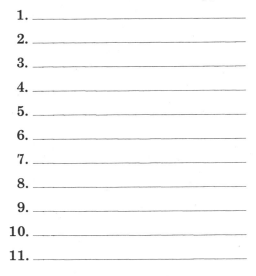

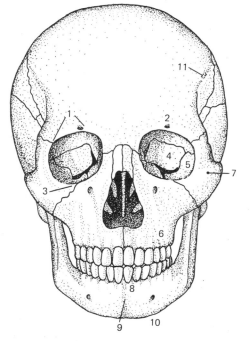

Supplemental Structures of Dental Importance—Lateral View

The information below describes and locates structures either on or in the skull that are important to dentistry.

Name	Location and Description
Nasion (nā′-ze-on)	A slight depression at the root of the nose marking the midpoint of the frontonasal suture.
Glabella (glà-bel′-ah)	The smooth prominence between the superciliary ridges (eyebrows).
Anterior nasal spine	A sharp process at the anterior superior portion of the maxillae. It is on the midline.
Zygomatic arches	Parts of the temporal bones—the arches of bone, one on each side of the skull; they unite the malar bones and the temporal bones by an oblique suture.
External acoustical meatus	The openings of the natural passages into the ears. They are located on the temporal bones.
Mastoid processes	Conical projections on the inferior surfaces of the temporal bones, posterior to the external acoustical meatus. They serve as attachments for various muscles.
Styloid processes	Slender, pointed bones that project downward and forward from the inferior surface of the temporal bones. They serve as attachments for various muscles and ligaments.
Glenoid fossae	Smooth depressions on the inferior surface of the temporal bones, and anterior to the external acoustical meatus. They articulate with the mandibular condyles to form the temporomandibular joint.
Occipital protuberance	The most posterior bony prominence in the midline at the junction of the head and the neck. It is located on the occipital bone.
Occipital condyles	Posterior inferior oval convexities on either side of the foramen magnum.
Lambdoidal suture	The interlocking line between the parietal and the occipital bones.
Lambda (lam′-dah)	The meeting point of the lambdoidal and the sagittal sutures.

NEW WORDS

Acoustical (à-kōos′-ti-kal): Pertaining to acoustics; serving to aid hearing.

Fossa (fos′-à): A pit or depression.

Process: Any marked prominence or projecting part; an outgrowth or extension.

Protuberance: A projection or prominence.

Meatus (mē-ā′-tus): A natural opening or passage (*meatus* is both singular and plural in form).

Articulate: To unite by a joint.

Study the illustration below and then take the Self-Test on the page that follows.

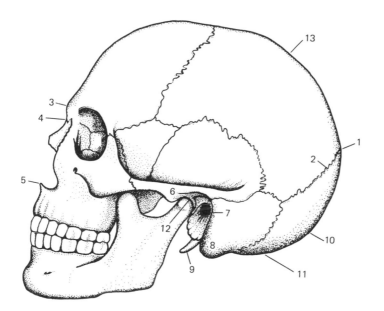

Supplemental structures of dental importance (lateral view). (1) Lambda; (2) lambdoidal suture; (3) glabella; (4) nasion; (5) anterior nasal spine; (6) zygomatic arch; (7) acoustical meatus; (8) mastoid process; (9) styloid process; (10) occipital protuberance; (11) occipital condyles; (12) glenoid fossa; (13) sagittal suture.

SELF—TEST

Write in the names of the supplemental structures on the lines provided below.

1. _____

2. _____

3. _____

4. _____

5. _____

6. _____

7. _____

8. _____

9. _____

10. _____

11. _____

12. _____

13. _____

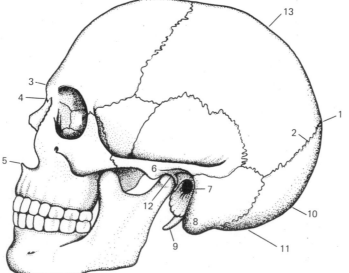

There are two maxillae: one right and one left, forming the bulk of the upper jaw. They are joined in the roof of the mouth (palate) by a suture known as the *intermaxillary suture*, the *median palatine suture*, or the *palatine raphe*. All of these terms are correct. There are four processes on the maxillae, some of which are paired; and there are four foramen. Three foramen are paired and the fourth (the incisive) has one opening; however, two lateral canals can be seen. The functions of the maxillae are to give shape to the face, to form part of the eyesocket and the nasal cavity, to support the upper teeth, to form the palate, and to hold the maxillary sinus (also known as the *antrum of Highmore*).

Processes and Foramina

There are several processes and foramina in the maxillae. The processes will be discussed first. The numbers of parts are shown in parentheses.

Processes	*Location and Description*
Frontal (nasal) (1)	A strong, irregular process that stands vertically above the body of the maxillae proper and forms part of the lateral boundaries of the nose. The superior part articulates with the frontal bone and the lateral part with the nasal bones.
Malar (zygomatic) (2)	A rough triangular process that articulates with the malar bone to form the cheek bone.
Palatine (2)	This process forms the anterior three-fourths of the hard palate or roof of the mouth. The remaining fourth is formed by a portion of the palatine bones.
Alveolar (1)	The alveolar process consists of two compact bony plates joined together by interdental septa, thus forming sockets for the teeth. It is the portion of the jaw that surrounds and supports the maxillary teeth.

Foramina	*Location and Description*
Incisive	The incisive foramen lies immediately behind the central incisors on the midline. It is sometimes known as the *nasopalatine foramen*. This foramen has two lateral canals in the opening. The dentist, in order to anesthetize, will insert the needle immediately laterally to the incisive papilla, directing it upward, slightly medially, and backward. This injection of the anterior one-third of the palate anesthetizes the mucoperiosteum, giving anesthesia to the centrals, laterals, and canines on either side of the midline. Usually a partial palatine injection is also needed for anesthesia in the canine area.

Foramina	Location and Description
Posterior palatine (2)	These formamina are also called the *greater* or the *major palatine foramina*. They lie at the level of the distal half of the last molars about 3/16 inch (4 mm) anterior to the posterior border of the hard palate. The dentist will insert the needle at the height of the curving arch, directing it upward, backward, and outward. This injection will anesthetize the mucoperiosteum of the palate from the tuberosity to the canine region and from the median line to the gingival crest on the side injected.
Posterior superior alveolar (2)	These foramina are situated directly superior to the disto-gingival margin of the maxillary third molar.
Infraorbital (2)	The infraorbital foramina are situated 1/4 to 3/8 inch (8 to 10 mm) below the middle part of the inferior orbital rim, and near the upper and inner corners of the canine fossae. The dentist will locate the foramen by palpation. The needle is introduced into the infraorbital canal. Anesthesia will be obtained in the incisors, canines, premolars, and the mesio-buccal root of the first molar, as well as in associated structures.

NEW WORDS

Mucoperiosteum (mu'-ko-per"-e-os'-te-um): Periosteum having a mucous surface.

Palpation (pal-pā'-shun): Feeling with the fingers or hand to determine by use of the tactile senses the physical characteristics of tissues or organs.

Periosteum (per"-ē-os'-tē-um): A specialized connective tissue covering all bones of the body. It possesses bone-forming potential and serves as attachment for certain muscles.

Septum: A wall or partition dividing a body space or cavity. Some septa are membranous; some are composed of bone; some are composed of cartilage.

Study the processes and foramina as illustrated; cover them and then take the Self-Test below.

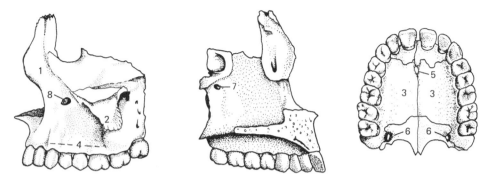

The Processes and Foramina of the Maxillae. Processes: (1) frontal (nasal); (2) malar (zygomatic); (3) palatine; (4) alveolar. Foramina: (5) incisive; (6) posterior palatine; (7) posterior superior alveolar; (8) infraorbital.

SELF—TEST

Write in the names of the processes and foramina of the maxillae on the lines provided below.

Processes

1. _____

2. _____

3. _____

4. _____

Foramina

5. _____

6. _____

7. _____

8. _____

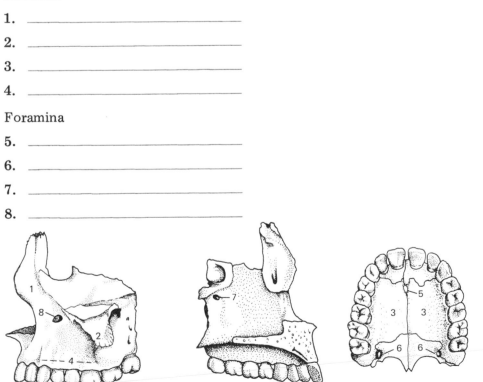

Supplemental Structures of the Maxillae

The information below describes and locates important structures on the maxillae.

Structure	Location and Description
Posterior nasal spine	The posterior nasal spine is formed by the joining of the horizontal portions of the palatine bones, which end in a sharp spine at the midline of the palate.
Median palatine suture	The median palatine suture is the suture marking the site of the joining of the maxillary bones during embryological development.
Incisive suture	The incisive suture is the site of joining between the premaxillae and the maxillary palatine processes.
Transverse palatine suture	The transverse palatine suture marks the site of joining between the maxillary palatine processes and the horizontal portions of the palatine bones.
Pterygoid hamulus	The pterygoid processes of the sphenoid bone are divided into medial and lateral plates. At the inferior end of the medial plate is a thin sharp bone known as the *pterygoid hamulus*. This bone is separated from the maxillary tuberosity by a deep notch known as the *hamular notch*.
Maxillary tuberosities	The maxillary tuberosities are the most posterior, rounded eminences on the maxillae. They are located on both right and left just posterior to the last molar. They are most prominent after the third molars have completed their growth.

Study the illustrations below and then take the Self-Test on the page that follows.

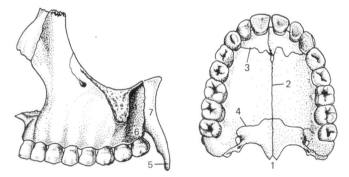

Supplementary structures of dental importance of the maxillae. (1) Posterior nasal spine; (2) median palatine suture; (3) incisive suture; (4) transverse palatine suture; (5) pterygoid hamulus; (6) maxillary tuberosity; (7) medial plate of the pterygoid process of the sphenoid.

SELF—TEST

Write in the names of the supplementary structures of the maxillae on the lines provided below.

1. _____

2. _____

3. _____

4. _____

5. _____

6. _____

7. _____

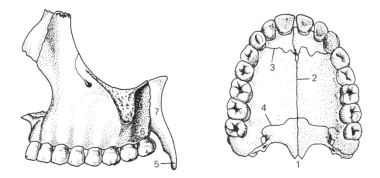

The Paranasal Sinuses

The eight paranasal sinuses are: (1) the maxillary sinuses in the body of the maxillae; (2) the frontal sinuses in the frontal bone; (3) the sphenoid sinuses in the sphenoid bone, and (4) the ethmoid sinuses in the ethmoid bone. The ethmoid sinuses differ somewhat from the others as they are composed of many small thin-walled cavities.

The Maxillary Sinuses. The maxillary sinuses are of particular importance to the dental auxiliary as the roots of the upper premolars and molars lie close to the floor of these sinuses; at best, the roots are separated from the sinus by only a thin layer of spongy bone. Sometimes even this layer of bone is missing, and then the root ends are covered only by mucous membrane; therefore, infections may spread rapidly. All maxillary extractions are carried out with care lest traumatic sinusitis result, or lest a root tip be pushed into the antrum (cavity).

A sinus infection produces symptoms that might cause the patient to question the health of the underlying maxillary teeth, because the infection can often be accompanied by tenderness of some or all of the upper teeth.

It is also important that you, as a dental auxiliary, recognize the location of the maxillary sinus, as you must not confuse its appearance in a radiograph with an abscess or other abnormality. You should be aware that the size of the maxillary sinus will vary among individuals, not reaching its full size until after the permanent dentition has erupted. If a tooth is lost, the sinus will often dip down into the space almost to the crest of the alveolar process.

Study the illustrations below and then take the Self-Test on the page that follows.

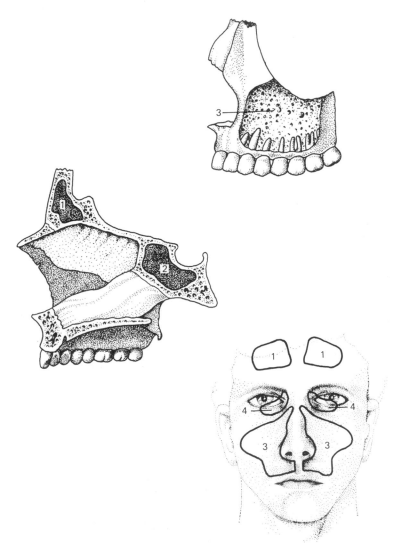

The paranasal sinuses. (1) Frontal [2]; (2) sphenoid [2]; (3) maxillary [2]; (4) ethmoid [2].

SELF—TEST

Write in the names of the four paranasal sinuses on the lines provided below.

1. _____

2. _____

3. _____

4. _____

79

The mandible is a strong, horseshoe-shaped bone lying below the maxillae. It consists of a body, two rami (upright processes on either side of the jaw bone), five processes (two condyloid, two coronoid, and one alveolar), and two paired foramina. The functions of the mandible are to give shape to the lower part of the face, to form the framework for the floor of the mouth, and to support the lower teeth.

Processes and Foramina

There are several processes and foramina on the mandible. The processes will be discussed first.

Processes	Location and Description
Condyloid (2)	The condyloid processes are located on the posterior superior portions of the two rami. Their purpose is to form the temporomandibular articulation between the temporal bones of the skull and the mandible. These processes fit into the glenoid fossae (mandibular fossae) of the temporal bones. On the anterior surfaces of the condyloid processes, there are depressions that form a place of attachment for the lateral pterygoid muscles.
Coronoid (2)	The coronoid processes are located on the anterior superior portions of each ramus. The external surfaces give attachment to the masseter muscle, and the medial surfaces serve as attachments for the deep tendon of the temporal muscle.
Alveolar (1)	The alveolar process consists of two compact bony plates joined together by interdental septa, thus forming sockets for the teeth. This process composes the superior border of the body of the mandible.

Foramina	Location and Description
Mandibular (2)	The mandibular foramina are situated on the lingual aspect of the upright portions of the mandible. In order to accomplish anesthesia, the dentist will palpate the retromolar fossa, place the syringe between the premolars on the opposite side, and deposit the anesthetic in the area of the mandibular foramen. Anesthesia will usually be obtained in all of the teeth up to, but not including, the central and lateral teeth on the side injected, as these teeth may receive innervation from overlapping nerve fibers from the opposite side.
Mental (2)	The mental foramina are the openings into the mental canals. They are situated in a vertical plane on the facial

Foramina	Location and Description
	side of the mandible between and inferior to the premolars. This injection may be used when a complete block is unnecessary or contraindicated. It will anesthetize the premolars and canines.

Study the illustration; cover it and then take the Self-Test below.

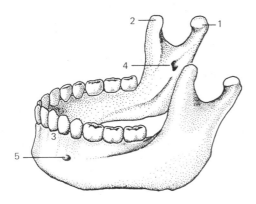

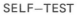

The mandibular processes and foramina. (1) Condyloid process [2]; (2) coronoid process [2]; (3) alveolar process [1]; (4) mandibular foramen [2]; (5) mental foramen [2].

SELF—TEST

Write in the names of the processes and the foramina of the mandible on the lines provided below.

1. _____

2. _____

3. _____

4. _____

5. _____

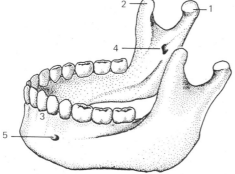

Supplemental Structures of the Mandible.

The definitions below describe and locate supplemental structures on the mandible that are of dental importance.

Structure	Location and Description
Mylohyoid line	This line (ridge) is found lingually on either side of the symphysis. It extends posteriorly and gives rise to the mylohyoid muscle as well as other structures. This structure is sometimes called the *internal oblique ridge*.
Retromolar triangle	This triangle is located behind the last molar on both sides of the mandible. It is a continuation of the coronoid process that widens as it progresses downward to form a bony triangle. The medial and lateral surfaces of this triangle extend forward to the buccal and the lingual of the third molar area.
Genial tubercle	Sometimes called the *mental spine*. It is located on the lingual and slightly above the border of the mandible at the midline. It consists of several sharp spines surrounding a small foramen. It serves as the origin of the geniohyoid muscles.
Lingual foramen	This foramen is a very small foramen in the center of the mental spine. It supplies innervation to the lingual mucosa and possibly some to the plexus in the incisor area.
Mandibular notch	This notch separates the coronoid and the condyloid processes. It is sometimes called the *sigmoid notch*.
External oblique ridge	This ridge is also known as the *oblique line*. It is a strong ridge that is continuous with the anterior border of the coronoid process. It diminishes as it goes forward toward the mental tubercles. It affords attachment for muscles.
Angle of the jaw	The angle is where the body of the mandible and the posterior border of the ramus meet.
Rami	The rami are the upright portions of the mandible.

Study the illustrations below; then take the Self-Test on the page that follows.

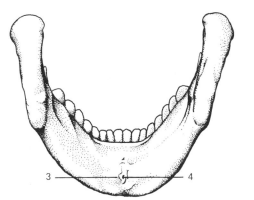

Mandible: Posterior aspect

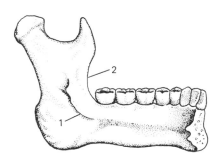

The left half of the mandible:
Medial aspect

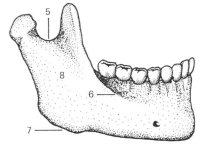

The right half of the mandible:
Lateral aspect

Supplemental structures of the mandible. (1) Mylohyoid line; (2) retromolar triangle; (3) genial tubercle; (4) lingual foramen; (5) mandibular notch; (6) external oblique ridge; (7) angle of the jaw; (8) rami.

Write in the names of the supplementary structures of the mandible on the
lines provided below.

1. _____

2. _____

3. _____

4. _____

5. _____

6. _____

7. _____

8. _____

Mandible: Posterior aspect

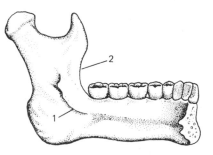

The left half of the mandible:
Medial aspect

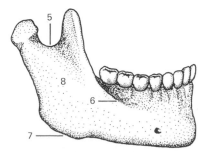

The right half of the mandible:
Lateral aspect

The Temporomandibular Joint. The *TMJ*, as the temporomandibular joint is known, is the joint that permits a wide range of motion to the mandible. It derives its name from the two bones that form the joint: the temporal bone and the condyle of the mandible. As with all joints, there are ligaments, cartilage, and synovial membrane to provide movement. The depression in the temporal bone in which the condyle of the mandible rests is called the *glenoid fossa.*

The temporomandibular joint of the human body is the only joint that can be dislocated without the action of external force. Displacement is always anterior. To reduce the dislocation, the pull of the spastic muscles must be overcome by a strong downward pressure. Then the mandible glides easily backward into its correct position.[1]

Some common causes for TMJ disorders are: (1) overclosure of the mandible; (2) occlusal disharmonies, and (3) mental tension.[2] An important symptom of temporomandibular joint disorder is pain in the region—pain that radiates into the temple, the ear, the throat, the cheek, and the tongue.[3] One of the most common disorders is called *tic douloureux*, which is trigeminal neuralgia.

Study the parts of the temporomandibular joint as illustrated and then take the Self-Test on the page that follows.

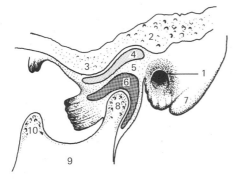

Parts of the temporomandibular joint. (1) External acoustical meatus or auditory canal; (2) glenoid fossa or mandibular fossa or articular fossa—all are correct; (3) articular eminence or tubercle; (4) superior synovial cavity (filled with synovial fluid that is similar to egg white); (5) meniscus or articular disk (fibrous cartilage); (6) inferior synovial cavity; (7) mastoid process; (8) mandibular condyle; (9) ramus; (10) mandibular coronoid process.

[1]Sicher, *Oral Anatomy*, 4th ed (St. Louis, Mo.: The C. V. Mosby Co., 1965), p. 501.

[2]Ibid, p. 496.

[3]Ibid, p. 497.

Write in the names of the parts of the temporomandibular joint on the lines provided.

1. _____

2. _____

3. _____

4. _____

5. _____

6. _____

7. _____

8. _____

9. _____

10. _____

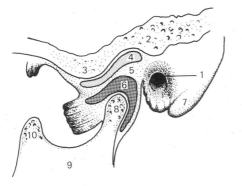

Pharynx, Larynx, and Trachea. The following information is presented to reinforce what was learned in the section on the Respiratory System contained in Chapter 1.

The pharynx is divided into three parts as listed below, and serves not only as a passageway for air but also as a passageway for the food we eat.

1. The nasopharynx (na″-zo-far′-inks) is the upper portion of the pharynx that lies immediately behind the nasal cavity. Located on the posterior wall of the nasopharynx is the pharyngeal tonsil (adenoid).

2. The oropharynx (o″-ro-far′-inks) forms the posterior wall of the fauces (the passageway from the mouth to the pharynx). On the lateral walls are found the palatine tonsils.

3. The laryngeal pharynx (lah-rin′-je-al) is the lower portion of the pharynx. This portion opens into two spaces. One space is to allow air to reach the larynx (lar′-inks), or voice box, and the other is to allow food to pass dorsally and on to the esophagus.

The action of swallowing (deglutition) brings the larynx against the epiglottis, which folds over the opening, allowing food to pass on to the esophagus with only an occasional mixup.

Study the parts of the pharynx, larynx, and trachea as illustrated and then take the Self-Test on the page that follows.

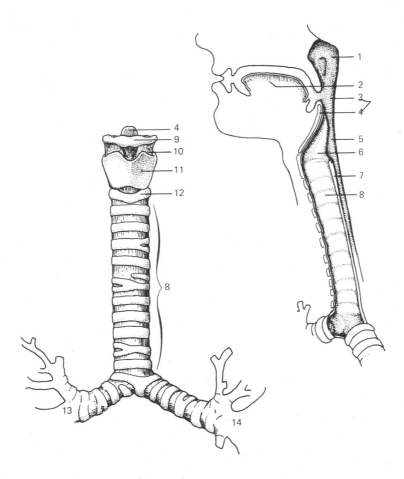

Parts of the pharynx, larynx, and trachea. (1) Nasopharynx; (2) tongue; (3) oropharynx; (4) epiglottis; (5) laryngeal pharynx; (6) larynx; (7) esophagus; (8) trachea; (9) hyoid bone; (10) thyrohyoid membrane; (11) thyroid cartilage; (12) cricoid cartilage; (13) right bronchus; (14) left bronchus.

Write in the names of the parts of the pharynx, larynx, and trachea on the lines provided.

1. _____   8. _____

2. _____   9. _____

3. _____   10. _____

4. _____   11. _____

5. _____   12. _____

6. _____   13. _____

7. _____   14. _____

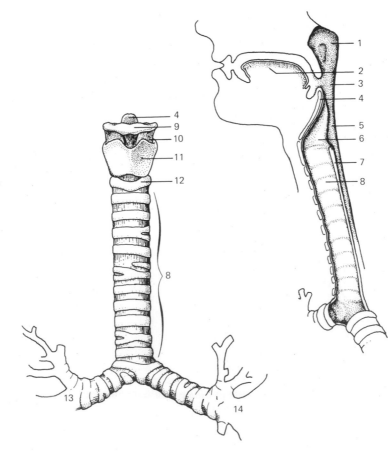

The Hyoid Bone. The hyoid bone is important because it forms the attachment for the hyoid muscles and ligaments. it consists of three parts: the body (single), and the greater and lesser horns or *cornua* (hornlike projections).

The hyoid bone is a rather small U-shaped bone placed in the upper part of the neck at the median line, near the base of the tongue, and extending posteriorly. It is sometimes called the *skeleton of the tongue.* It has no bony connection with other bones, and so it is classified as a floating bone.

Study the parts of the hyoid bone as illustrated; cover the illustration and take the Self-Test below.

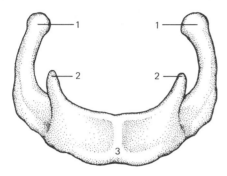

Parts of the hyoid bone. (1) Greater cornua; (2) lesser cornua; (3) body.

SELF—TEST

Write in the names of the three parts of the hyoid bone on the lines provided below.

1. _____

2. _____

3. _____

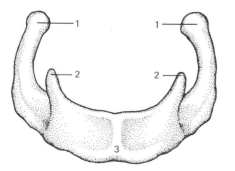

The mouth, or *oral cavity*, is a cavity bound anteriorly and laterally by the lips and cheeks; posteriorly, it communicates with the oropharynx. Superiorly, the roof is formed by the hard and soft palate; and inferiorly, the floor is formed by the sublingual region under the tongue. The cavity contains primarily the tongue, the orifices of ducts, the salivary glands, and the teeth. The space between the lips and the teeth and between the cheeks and the teeth is called the *vestibule* or the *vestibular fornix*. The cavity that is filled with the tongue is called the *cavity proper*.

The following definitions describe and locate structures in and around the oral cavity that are of dental importance.

Structure	Location and Description
Hard palate	The hard palate is the anterior two-thirds of the palate. It is sometimes referred to as the *roof of the mouth*. It is formed by the joining of the two palatine processes of the maxillae at the midline. It is covered with keratinized mucosa. Beneath the mucosa, in most areas, is submucosa containing the larger blood vessels and nerves.
Incisive papilla	The incisive papilla is a fleshy prominence immediately posterior to the maxillary incisors and on the midline. It marks the opening to the incisive canal.
Rugae (roo'-je)	The rugae are also found on the hard palate just lingual to the central incisors. They appear as transverse ridges of dense fibrous tissue. The rugae of the hard palate are aptly named, as the word *rugae* means "wrinkles" or "folds."
Soft palate	The soft palate is the remaining one-third of the palate. It extends posteriorly from the hard palate. It is covered with mucosa; however, this mucosa is not keratinized. It is lining mucosa similar to that found under the tongue and lining the cheeks and the lips. At the midline of the soft palate and on the lower posterior border is a fingerlike conical process called the *palatine uvula*. This muscular tissue guards the opening from the nasal cavity and the upper pharynx, preventing foods and liquids from entering the nasal cavities during the process of swallowing.
Palatal fovea	Between the hard and soft palate, close to the midline, can often be seen a small depression or depressions (the palatal fovea). These depressions represent the openings to ducts that lead from the palatal salivary glands.
Pterygomandibular raphe (ter"-i-go-man-dib'-u-lar ra'-fe)	The raphe is a band of tendinous tissue extending down from the hamular area (just posterior to the maxillary tuberosities), to the retromolar pads on the mandible on both right and left.
Frena	The frena are triangular pieces of tissue that hold, in the oral cavity, the lips to the mucosa and the tongue to the

Structure	*Location and Description*
Frena (continued)	floor of the mouth. Only three will be discussed: two labial and one lingual. The *lingual frenum* is sometimes very short, causing a tongue-tied condition. The *maxillary labial frenum* is the strongest. It sometimes will grow down between the central incisors causing a diastema. The *mandibular frenum* is sometimes absent; then again it may be so large that it will cause a periodontal condition or interfere with the placing of dentures. The type of surgery done to correct these problems is called a *frenectomy*.
Tongue	The tongue (glossa) is a very strong muscular organ that aids in chewing and swallowing and, in addition, is one of the principal organs of speech. The Latin word *lingua* meaning "tongue" gave rise to our word *language*. Dividing the dorsal surface of the tongue into two equal halves is the *median septum* or midline, and on this surface are a number of special organs called *taste buds* (papillae). These organs are actually groups of modified epithelial cells with the ability to respond to certain substances, giving us our sense of taste. The mucosa covering the dorsal surface of the tongue is called *specialized mucosa*.
Papillae	The largest of the papillae on the tongue's dorsal surface are the *circumvallate papillae*. They are located to the posterior of the dorsal surface of the tongue. They are large, round, doughnut-shaped elevations arranged in an upside down "V" on both sides of the midline. The *filiform papillae* are tall hairlike, cone-shaped elevations. These papillae are the most numerous of the papillae. they cover the entire dorsal surface of the tongue anterior to the vallate papillae, giving the tongue a velvety appearance. The *fungiform papillae* are distributed between the filiform, and they appear as small single mushroomlike elevations. They are dark red in color, therefore easily distinguished from the filiform papillae. The *foliate papillae* are on the posterior lateral borders of the tongue; they appear as low parallel folds. They may be seen by grasping the tongue with a gauze square, gently pulling it outward, and turning it to one side and then to the other. It is at times difficult to find them, for frequently they are almost nonexistent. They too are the site of taste buds. All of the papillae tend to collect debris. Therefore, to keep the tongue clean, it is wise to brush this area gently each time the teeth are brushed.
Labial commissures	A *commissure* may be defined as a band of fibers joining corresponding opposite parts. The labial commissures are the corners of the mouth where the lips meet.
Fauces	The *fauces* is the name given to the passage leading from the mouth into the pharynx. On either side of the fauces there are two sets of arches that mark the outline of the

Structure	Location and Description
Fauces (continued)	fauces. (1) The *anterior arches* are known by several names: the *glossopalatine arches*, *palatoglossal folds*, *anterior tonsilar pillars*, or *anterior pillars*. (2) The *posterior arches* also have many names: the *pharyngopalatine arches*, *palatopharyngeal folds*, *posterior tonsilar pillars*, or *posterior pillars*.
Palatine tonsils	The palatine tonsils are usually found as two large masses of lymphoid tissue situated on either side of the fauces in the triangular space between the glossopalatine and the pharyngopalatine arches. The palatine tonsils, if present, are visible when the mouth is held open and the tongue is pulled forward and depressed slightly with a tongue blade.
Foramen caecum (sē'-kum)	At the most posterior area of the tongue, in the midline, is the foramen caecum, which appears as a deep depression.
Lingual tonsil	On the lateral and most posterior surface of the tongue is a mass of lymphoid tissue known as the *lingual tonsil*. This mass of tissue along with the adenoids (nasopharyngeal tonsils) and the palatine tonsils form the so-called Waldeyer's ring, a ring that is one of nature's protective devices.
Sublingual fold	This fold of tissue is found under the tongue. It extends from either side of the lingual frenum, marking the site of the sublingual salivary glands. On the superior surface can at times be seen the openings to the *ducts of Rivinus*, minor ducts inferior to the tongue and on the superior surface of the sublingual gland. These ducts open at the crest of the sublingual eminence on the floor of the oral cavity.
Salivary caruncula (kah-rung'-ku-lah)	The salivary caruncula is a small fleshy eminence at the midline and close to the lingual frenum. This eminence, or papilla, marks the site where the ducts of the sublingual and submandibular salivary glands join to empty saliva into the oral cavity.
Fimbriated folds (fim'-brē-āted)	These irregular, fringed folds of tissue are found on the inferior lateral surface of the tongue. They extend in an oblique fashion on either side of the midline from anterior to posterior.
Gingiva	The gingiva is the keratinized tissue surrounding the teeth. When in good health, it appears as firm, pink, and stippled tissue. Just inferior to the gingiva is the mucosa, which appears soft, shiny, and dark pink due to the rich blood supply in this area. The junction where the gingiva and the mucosa meet is called the *mucogingival border*.
Lips	We, as humans, have something that is individual with us— the lips: no other animal has these organs. The red part of the lip is a zone of nonkeratinized, very thin epithelium covering a rich capillary supply. It is called the *vermilion*

Structure	Location and Description
	border. The protruding portion at the midline of the upper lip is called the *labial tubercle.*
Nasolabial groove	The nasolabial groove occurs on both sides of the nose. It separates the lips from the cheeks. It extends from the ala, the rounded eminences on either side of the nose, downward in an oblique fashion, ending some distance lateral to the labial commissures. It is not seen in the very young. As one grows older, this groove deepens.
Philtrum	The philtrum is a shallow depression extending from the nose to the upper lip. It is on the midline. It marks the joining of these parts during the embryological stage of development.
Labiomental groove	The labiomental groove is just inferior to the lower lip. It is a horizontal groove that separates the lip from the chin. This groove, like the nasolabial groove, deepens with age.
Ranine vein	This vein begins near the tip of the inferior surface of the tongue. It is a large vein.
Mucosa	The mucosa is a membrane covered with epithelium that lines canals and cavities communicating with the exterior of the body. In the oral cavity it lines the lips, cheeks, under the tongue, the soft palate, and the vestibule to the mucogingival border. It is the site of numerous salivary minor glands.

Taste Sensations

Some of the sensations we call *taste* actually are smells detected by the olfactory organs in the nose. When one has a cold or holds his nose, while tasting food, it is difficult to distinguish some flavors. The sense of taste may also be stimulated or altered by chemical and natural means. Ice can also be used to destroy taste temporarily. At times, in older persons, taste tends to deteriorate, and sometimes illness may destroy or alter taste. There are primarily four taste sensations: sweet, sour (acid), salty, and bitter.

Study the structures of the oral cavity as illustrated and then take the Self-Test on the page that follows.

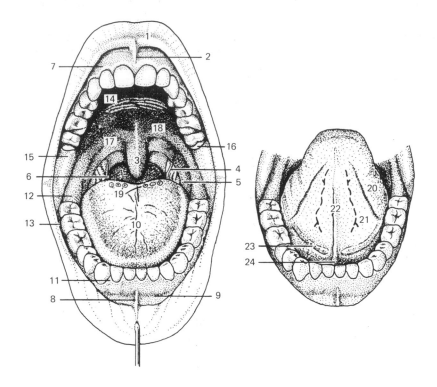

Parts of the oral cavity. (1) Lip or vermilion border; (2) labial frenum, maxillary; (3) uvula; (4) tonsil, palatine; (5) glossopalatine arch; (6) pharyngopalatine arch; (7) gingiva; (8) labial frenum, mandibular; (9) mucogingival border; (10) tongue midline; (11) interdental papilla; (12) retromolar pad; (13) vestibule; (14) rugae; (15) pterygomandibular raphe; (16) maxillary tuberosity; (17) soft palate; (18) hard palate; (19) circumvallate papillae; (20) plica fimbriate or fimbriated folds; (21) ranine vein; (22) lingual frenum; (23) sublingual fold; (24) salivary caruncula.

SELF—TEST

Write in the names of the oral cavity structures on the lines provided.

1. _____   13. _____

2. _____   14. _____

3. _____   15. _____

4. _____   16. _____

5. _____   17. _____

6. _____   18. _____

7. _____   19. _____

8. _____   20. _____

9. _____   21. _____

10. _____   22. _____

11. _____   23. _____

12. _____   24. _____

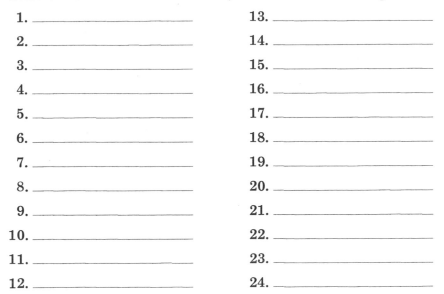

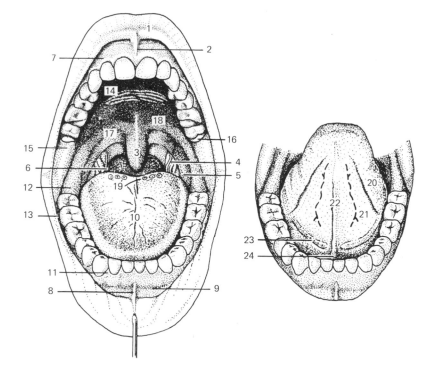

The Salivary Glands

The sight or smell of food—even the thought of food—will at times promote the flow of saliva from the salivary glands. Saliva is mostly water, containing minerals, trace elements, enzymes, and amino acids among other things. This wonderful fluid has many functions other than the moistening of food for easier swallowing—such as improving the sense of taste, providing partial digestion of some starchy foods, helping to keep the teeth and mouth clean, aiding in the maintanance of body water balance, enhancing antibacterial action, and providing a buffering capacity that reduces the rate of dental caries. Three pairs of major salivary glands plus many minor glands, produce from 1 to 3 pints of saliva daily to perform all of these functions.

Salivary stones will occasionally result in blockage in the area of the salivary ducts, causing swelling and tenderness, a condition that of course may also result from infections. However, if the swelling is caused by blockage, it will fluctuate, especially at mealtimes. Occasionally surgery is required to remove a stone from the duct.

Dry mouth is another very disturbing problem. This can be caused by many things. There are two drugs that can cause this condition—atropine and morphine. Vitamin B deficiency and aging may also be factors.

The following describes and locates the major and minor salivary glands associated with the oral cavity.

Major Salivary Glands	Location and Description
Parotid glands	The parotid glands are the largest of the salivary glands. They lie in front of and slightly below the ears. The secretion from these glands is watery, or serous, and it is discharged into the oral cavity by way of the parotid duct, or Stenson's duct. The opening of this duct is marked by a raised tab of tissue called the *parotid papilla*. This papilla lies approximately opposite the maxillary second molar on the inner surface of the cheek. The papilla may be felt with the tongue or may be seen by looking into someone's mouth. Because of the calcium and phosphorous in saliva and because of the location of this duct, one of the heaviest deposits of calculus will be found on the buccal surface of the maxillary second molar. Parotid glands are the ones affected when mumps, a highly infectious disease, is present.
Submandibular glands	The submandibular glands are also known as the *submaxillary glands*. Either name is correct. Originally they were called the submaxillary because of their location below the maxillary bones. These glands lie beneath the lower jaw on either side. The secretion from these glands is sticky and mixed. They discharge their secretion by way of the submandibular duct, or Wharton's duct, which opens into the floor of the mouth at the midline just lingual to the mandibular incisors. These glands are about the size of a walnut.

Major Salivary Glands	Location and Description
Submandibular glands (continued)	A heavy deposit of calculus will usually occur on the lingual of the central incisors because of the location of Wharton's duct.
Sublingual glands	The sublingual glands are long and flat; they lie beneath the tongue on either side. the secretion from these glands is thick and viscid. It is discharged into the oral cavity by way of Bartholin's duct, which either unites with or opens close to Wharton's duct at the midline. There is a lesser group of ducts, the ducts of Rivinus, that discharge some saliva into the sublingual area.

Minor Salivary Glands	Location and Description
Buccal	The buccal glands are located in the submucosa of the cheeks.
Palatine	These numerous glands are located primarily in the posterior part of the palate.
Labial	The labial glands are in the submucosa that lies beneath the mucosa on the inner surface of the lips. They can readily be seen by extending the lip and rolling it under.
	There are many other minor salivary glands that assist in keeping the oral cavity in a healthy condition.

Study the illustration of the salivary glands below and then take the Self-Test on the page that follows.

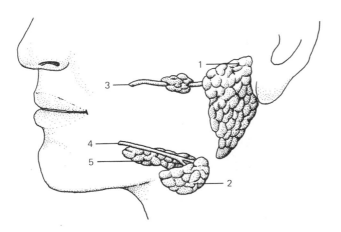

The salivary glands. (1) Parotid gland; (2) submandibular gland; (3) Stetson's duct; (4) Wharton's duct; (5) sublingual gland.

SELF—TEST

Write in the names of the salivary glands or ducts on the lines provided below.

1. _____

2. _____

3. _____

4. _____

5. _____

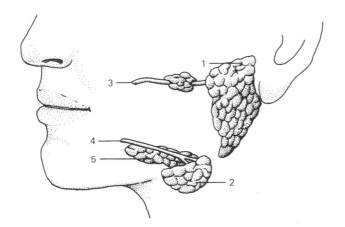

THE MUSCLES OF MASTICATION

There are generally believed to be three stages of mastication, which is the first act in the assimilation of food. These stages are: (1) the cutting or shearing of food; (2) the crushing of food into smaller particles, and (3) the grinding of food preparatory to deglutition.

When the neural impulse to masticate food is relayed along the muscles of mastication, the muscle fibers shorten, pulling toward their origin, and thus providing joint action. This reflex action permits the muscles of mastication to play a major role in preparing food for swallowing.

The teeth, also vital to the mastication of food, are generally arranged in both arches so that when the muscles of mastication bring the jaws together, the teeth meet in a functional relationship known as *occlusion*, with the maxillary and the mandibular teeth not quite in contact, but with a space of from 2 to 5 mm between the incisors. This is known as the *rest position*. Ideally the maxillary teeth overlap the mandibular teeth for a small fraction of an inch, with the maxillary teeth interdigitating with the mandibular teeth in order to function as a unit. This ideal relationship, or position, is known as the *centric position*.

Humans, being omnivorous (eating both meat and vegetable foods), have the ability to have an *eccentric* jaw position too. This means that certain muscles have the ability to move the mandible from side to side (lateral occlusion), as well as the ability to protract or retract the mandible.

The act of chewing, or mastication, consists of placing food between the anterior teeth and closing until the teeth meet with the mandibular incisors to the lingual of the maxillary incisors. Then with a shearing motion, a portion of food is cut free. The portion is then transferred by the tongue to the posterior teeth and is held in position by the cheeks and tongue. The inclined planes, ridges, and grooves of the opposing posterior teeth then reduce the food to bits. After the food has thus been prepared for deglutition, the tongue propels the bolus against the posterior of the palate and into the pharynx, and so on down the esophagus into the stomach.

There are hundreds of muscles associated with the head, neck, and face, but only a few will be discussed in this section.

NEW WORDS

Assimilation (ah-sim″-i-lā′-shun): Incorporation of nutritive material into the fluid or solid substance of the body.

Bolus (bo′-lus): A quantity of food entering the esophagus at one swallow.

The Buccinator Muscle

Study the information below and the illustration on the next page. Then cover the illustration and take the Self-Test that follows.

The buccinator muscle is the principal cheek muscle. It is considered an accessory muscle of mastication.

Form	Thin, flat quadrilateral (four-sided) muscle.
Position	Innermost muscle of the cheek.
Origin	Its fibers arise from the posterior lateral surfaces of the alveolar process of both maxillae and mandible, opposite the first, second, and third molars. The fibers in between arise from the pterygomandibular raphe. Stenson's (parotid) duct passes through this muscle opposite the second molar, to empty saliva into the oral cavity at the site of the parotid papilla.
Insertion	The fibers go forward to insert into other muscles that surround the mouth.
Function	This muscle compresses the cheek, expels air between the lips, and aids in the mastication of food.

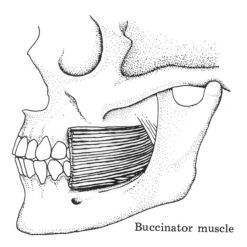

Buccinator muscle

SELF—TEST

Name this muscle and fill in the correct information after the words below.

1. Form: _____

2. Position: _____

3. Origin: _____

_____

_____

4. Insertion: _____

_____

5. Function: _____

Muscle: _____

The Masseter Muscle

Study the information below and the illustration on the next page. Then cover the illustration and take the Self-Test that follows.

The masseter (mah-sē′-ter) muscle is a powerful elevator muscle. It is so placed that, with the medial pterygoid, the mandible is suspended in a sling.

Form	Quadrilateral.
Position	Posterior on the lateral surface of the ramus.
Origin	It arises from the posterior one-third of the lower border of the zygomatic arch. The deep portion arises from the whole of the zygomatic arch to extend in an oblique fashion to the point of insertion.
Insertion	Lateral surface of the coronoid process of the mandible.
Function	It elevates the jaw, clenches the teeth, and brings the molar teeth together for crushing and grinding food. *Masseter* means "chewer."

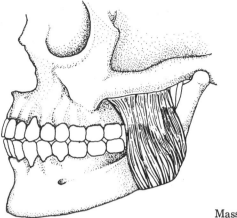

Masseter muscle.

SELF—TEST

Name this muscle and fill in the correct information after the word below:

1. Form: _____

2. Position: _____

3. Origin: _____

    _____

    _____

4. Insertion: _____

5. Function: _____

    _____

    Muscle: _____

The Medial Pterygoid Muscle

Study the information below and the illustration on the next page. Then cover the illustration and take the Self-Test that follows.

The medial pterygoid (ter'-i-goid) muscle is a powerful muscle but not as powerful as the masseter. This muscle and the masseter form a sling for the mandible.

Form	Flat and quadrilateral.
Position	Medial surface of the ramus.
Origin	The superior fibers extend downward in an oblique fashion from the pterygoid fossa and the medial surface of the lateral pterygoid plate, the pyramidal process of the palatine bone, and parts of the maxillary tuberosity.

Insertion   Lower posterior part of the medial surface of the ramus and the angle of the mandible.

Function   This muscle protracts and elevates the lower jaw; it assists in rotary motion while chewing.

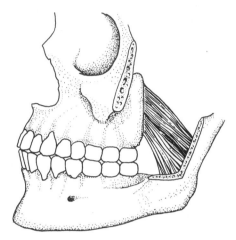

Medial (internal) pterygoid muscle.

SELF—TEST

Name this muscle and fill in the correct information after the words below.

1. Form: _____

2. Position: _____

3. Origin: _____

_____

_____

4. Insertion: _____

_____

5. Function: _____

_____

Muscle: _____

The Temporal Muscle

Study the information and illustration on the next page, then cover both and take the Self-Test.

The temporal muscle, unlike the masseter and the medial pterygoid muscle, is built for movement rather than power. It is primarily an elevator muscle.

Form	Fan-shaped.
Position	On the lateral surface of the skull.
Origin	Floor of the temporal fossa and the temporal facia (band of tissue).
Insertion	Into the coronoid process of the mandible and the anterior border of the ramus of the mandible.
Function	It elevates the jaw, retracts the mandible, and clenches the teeth.

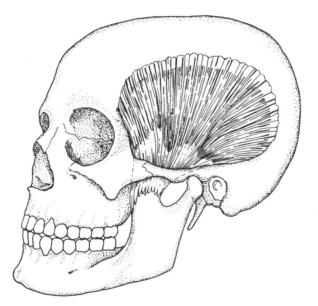

Temporal muscle.

SELF—TEST

Name this muscle and fill in the correct information after the words below.

1. Form: _____

2. Position: _____

3. Origin: _____

4. Insertion: _____

   _____

5. Function: _____

   Muscle: _____

The Lateral Pterygoid Muscle

Study the information and illustration below and then take the Self-Test that follows.

The lateral (external) pterygoid muscle is short and thick. It entends horizontally.

Form

Triangular with two heads: one is superior and one is inferior.

Position

On the lateral aspect of the skull.

Origin

The smaller superior head originates from the infratemporal surface of the greater wing of the sphenoid. The larger inferior head originates from the lateral pterygoid plate of the sphenoid bone.

Insertion

Anterior neck of the mandibular condyle and the articular disk where they fuse in front of the temporomandibular joint.

Function

Draws the mandible forward and rotates it downward and inward. It also assists in some lateral movement.

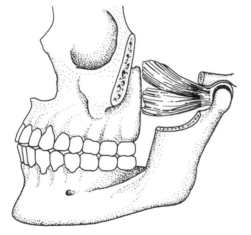

Lateral (external) pterygoid muscle.

SELF—TEST

Name this muscle and fill in the correct information after the words below.

1. Form: _____

2. Position: _____

3. Origin: _____

_____

4. Insertion: _____

_____

5. Function: _____

_____

Muscle: _____

The Orbicularis Oris Muscle

Study the information and illustration below and then take the Self-Test on the page that follows.

The orbicularis oris muscle is sometimes called the "kissing muscle" since it assists in the contraction of protrusion of the lips. This muscle is not attached to any of the skeleton bones. Some of its fibers come from other facial muscles.

Form	Circular.
Position	Surrounding the lips.
Origin	Formed by various facial muscles converging on the lips and by its own fibers.
Insertion	The fibers of this muscle interlace with each other at the midline.
Function	Compresses, contracts, and protrudes lips; assists in facial expression.

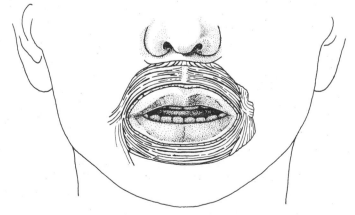

Orbicularis oris muscle.

SELF—TEST

Name this muscle and fill in the correct information after the words below.

1. Form: _____

2. Position: _____

3. Origin: _____

4. Insertion: _____

5. Function: _____

    Muscle: _____

Suprahyoid Muscles

    The suprahyoid muscles are not actually muscles of mastication, but they do assist by raising the hyoid bone and depressing the mandible during the mastication of food. The information following describes and locates additional muscles of dental importance.

Muscle	Location and Description
Mylohyoid	This is a flat, triangular muscle. It lies anterior and superior to the digastric muscle. It forms the floor of the mouth. This muscle has its origin from the entire mylohyoid line on the lingual surface of the mandible from the symphysis to the last molar. The posterior fibers insert into the hyoid bone, and the anterior fibers insert into the mylohyoid raphe. Its function is to raise the hyoid bone and the tongue.
Digastric	This muscle is a long, slender curved muscle that consists of two parts joined by a strong round tendon. It lies inferior to the mandible. The posterior portion arises from the mastoid notch of the temporal bone, which is found just medial to the mastiod process. It then passes anteriorly and inferiorly to the hyoid bone. The anterior portion arises from the digastric fossa on the inner side of the inferior border of the mandible and passes posteriorly and inferiorly to the hyoid bone. Neither the posterior or the anterior portion actually inserts into the hyoid bone, but both terminate at a round tendon that is held to the hyoid bone by a fibrous loop whose fibers are attached to the hyoid bone. This allows movement to both the anterior and the posterior portions. The function of this muscle is to raise the hyoid bone and move it forward and backward, and to assist other muscles in opening the jaws.
Geniohyoid	This muscle is long and slender. It lies superior to the mylohyoid muscle. It arises from the inferior mental spine (genio tubercles) on the inner surface of the mandible and inserts

Muscle	*Location and Function*
	into the hyoid bone. Its function is to draw the hyoid bone up and forward. It has some influence on drawing the tongue forward also.
Stylohyoid	This is a long slender muscle anterior and superior to the digastric muscle. It arises from the styloid process of the temporal bone and inserts into the hyoid bone. Its function is to draw the hyoid bone up and back.

Study the illustrations below and then take the Self-Test on the page that follows.

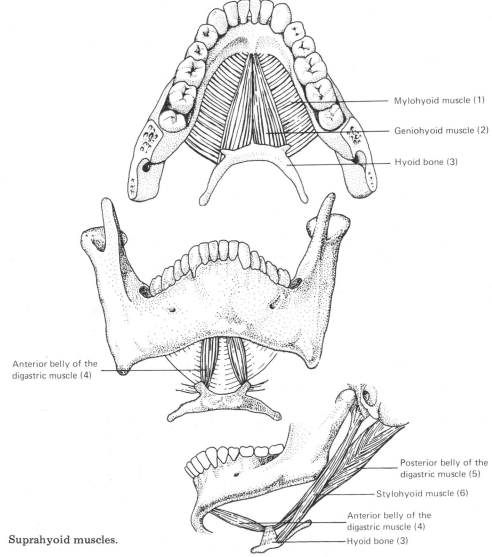

Mylohyoid muscle (1)

Geniohyoid muscle (2)

Hyoid bone (3)

Anterior belly of the digastric muscle (4)

Posterior belly of the digastric muscle (5)

Stylohyoid muscle (6)

Anterior belly of the digastric muscle (4)

Hyoid bone (3)

Suprahyoid muscles.

Write in the names of the suprahyoid muscles on the lines provided below.

1. _____

2. _____

3. _____

4. _____

5. _____

6. _____

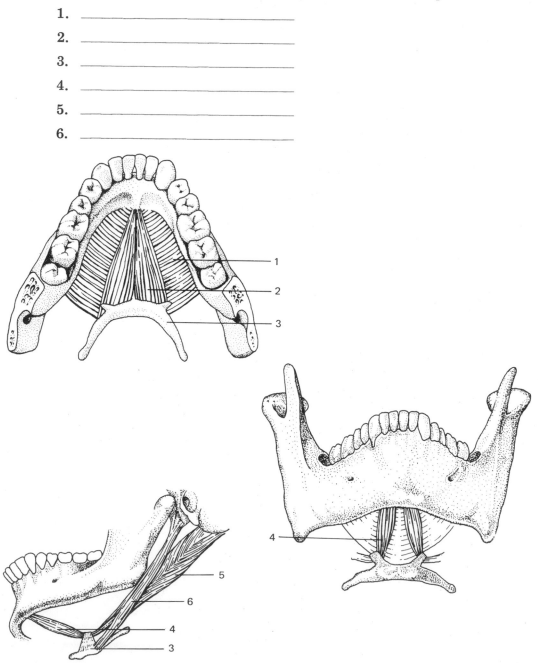

The fifth cranial nerve, or the trigeminal nerve, is often referred to as the "dental nerve" by those in the dental field, since two of its three branches are closely associated with the teeth and the surrounding structures.

This nerve emerges from the brain as a small motor root and a large sensory root. The motor root has its origin within the brain, while the sensory root has its origin in the Gasserion (semilunar) ganglion. The trigeminal nerve is a mixed nerve, as it furnishes both movement and sensation.

There are three main branches from the trigeminal nerve. Two branches are sensory, and one is both sensory and motor.

  I. Ophthalmic—sensory.
 II. Maxillary—sensory.
III. Mandibular—sensory and motor (mixed).

First Division: Ophthalmic Nerve

The ophthalmic nerve splits into three main branches immediately after leaving the orbit. The branches are as follows.

Nasociliary. The nasociliary branch furnishes sensation to the eyeball, the muscles controlling the eyeball, the anterior third of the nasal septum, and the lateral wall of the nasal cavity.

Frontal. The frontal branch furnishes sensation to the forehead, scalp, upper eyelid, frontal sinus, medial commissure of the eye, and root of the nose.

Lacrimal. The lacrimal branch furnishes sensation to the lacrimal gland, the conjunctiva, and the lateral commissure of the eye.

Second Division: Maxillary Nerve

The second division, or maxillary nerve, runs in a horizontal direction as it leaves the cranium by way of the foramen rotundum. It crosses the narrow pterygopalatine fossa and splits into three major branches, as described below.

Pterygopalatine. The pterygopalatine branch originates from the maxillary nerve with two short trunks that unite at the pterygopalatine ganglion, where it (the pterygopalatine nerve) then divides into four subbranches. (Note: The pterygopalatine ganglion is also known as the *sphenopalatine ganglion* and/or *Meckel's ganglion*.)

1. *Anterior palatine*: This subbranch descends through the posterior palatine canal and enters the oral cavity at the posterior palatine foramen. It then runs forward, together with the anterior palatine artery, in a special groove as far as the canine. This nerve innervates the hard

109

palate, the palatal alveolar plate, the periosteum, and the mucous membrane over the molars and premolars.

2. *Middle palatine*: This subbranch emerges from an accessory palatine foramen and innervates the soft palate, the uvula, and the upper portion of the palate.

3. *Posterior palatine*: This subbranch also emerges from an accessory palatine foramen; it innervates the soft palate and the tonsils.

4. *Nasopalatine*: This subbranch enters the oral cavity by way of the anterior (incisive) foramen; it serves the premaxillary bones, the lingual alveolar process, and the canines on either side. The two nasopalatine nerves extend posteriorly on either side of the palate as far as the canines, where they join with the anterior palatine nerves to form the inner loop.

Infraorbital. When the maxillary nerve enters the infraorbital canal, it becomes the infraorbital nerve, which continues through the infraorbital groove on the floor of the orbit and then forward in the infraorbital canal to finally emerge on the face at the infraorbital foramen. There are three subbranches from this nerve.

1. *Posterior superior alveolar*: This subbranch runs downward from the infraorbital, where it branches to pass through the apical foramina of the roots of the second and third molars, as well as through the lingual and distobuccal roots of the first molars. (Note: There is some difference of opinion as to whether this nerve originates directly from the maxillary nerve or from the infraorbital nerve.)

2. *Middle superior alveolar*: This subbranch runs downward to branch again and enter the apices of the upper premolars and the mesiobuccal roots of the first molars.

3. *Anterior superior alveolar*: This subbranch descends from the infraorbital nerve just before it emerges on the face. It serves the centrals, laterals, and canines with sensation.

The above nerves also furnish the periodontal ligaments, gingiva, interdental papilla, and the labial or buccal gingiva, surrounding the maxillary teeth with sensation. The terminal branches of the infraorbital nerve supply the lower eyelid, nose, and upper lip with sensation.

Zygomatic. The zygomatic nerve often appears to be a branch of the infraorbital nerve. It serves the lacrimal area and the skin over the height of the cheek. However, again, it is often considered a branch of the maxillary nerve as is the posterior superior alveolar nerve.

Third Division: Mandibular Nerve

The mandibular nerve is a mixed nerve. As the sensory root of the third division separates at the Gasserian ganglion (semilunar), it is joined by the motor root, with both dropping almost at right angles to enter the foramen oval to serve the muscles of mastication, the lower dentititon, and the surrounding tissues. This nerve also divides, and the three divisions of the sensory branch are described below.

Inferior Alveolar. The inferior alveolar branch, together with the inferior dental artery, passes through the mandibular foramen and transverses the mandibular canal in the body of the mandible, serving the alveolus of the molar teeth, the apices of the teeth, and the pulp. At the mental foramen the inferior alveolar nerve branches as follows:

1. *Mental nerve*: This branch emerges from the mental foramen to serve the skin of the chin, the lower lip from the mental foramen to the median line, and the labial mucosa inferior to the centrals and canines.
2. *Incisive nerve*: This nerve, a terminal branch of the inferior alveolar nerve, continues anteriorly to form a plexus that serves the alveoli and the pulps of the anterior teeth.

Lingual Nerve. The lingual nerve branches from the mandibular nerve to run downward anteriorly to the inferior alveolar nerve. It passes between the medial pterygoid muscle and the ascending ramus. Then it runs beneath the mucous membrane of the floor of the mouth near the apices of the lower third molar. It then goes internally toward the tongue, serving the anterior two-thirds of the tongue with sensation. It also innervates the lingual mucous membrane and the periosteum of all the lower teeth.

Buccal Nerve. The buccal nerve also branches from the mandibular nerve just outside the foramen oval. It passes between the two heads of the lateral pterygoid muscle and then anterior and buccal to the ramus to enter the buccinator muscle. The lowest branch of the buccal nerve, sometimes referred to as the long buccal nerve, supplies sensation to the buccal gingivae and mucosa.

Facial nerve. The facial nerve, or seventh cranial nerve, has two roots. The larger is the motor nerve to the muscles of facial expression. The smaller root supplies taste sensation to the anterior two-thirds of the tongue and general sensation to other areas in and around the head and neck.

NEW WORDS

Innervate (i′-nur-vāt): To supply with nerves.

Conjunctiva (kon″-junk-ti′-vah): The delicate membrane lining the eyelids and covering the eyeball.

Cutaneous (ku-tā′-ne-us): Pertaining to the skin.

Ganglion (gang′-gle-on): A group of nerve cell bodies.

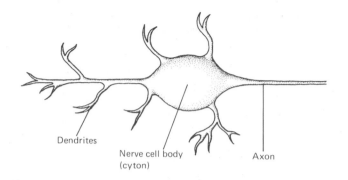

Dendrites

Nerve cell body
(cyton)

Axon

One type of neuron showing the various parts of the nerve cell.

Study the illustrations below and then take the Self-Test on the page that follows.

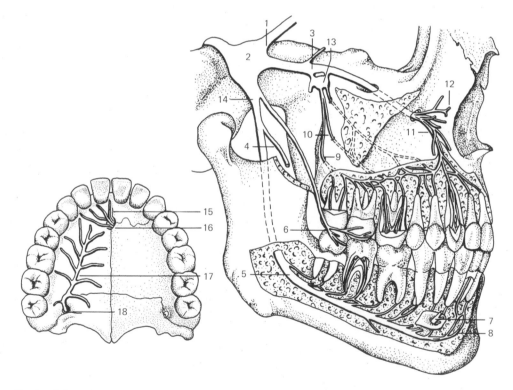

Parts of the trigeminal nerve. (1) Ophthalmic division; (2) gasserian ganglion; (3) maxillary division; (4) lingual nerve; (5) inferior alveolar nerve; (6) buccal nerve; (7) mental nerve; (8) incisive nerve; (9) posterior superior alveolar nerve; (10) middle superior alveolar nerve; (11) anterior superior alveolar nerve; (12) infraorbital nerve; (13) sphenopalatine ganglion (Meckle's ganglion); (14) mandibular division. The palatine nerves. (15) Nasopalatine nerve; (16) incisive foramen; (17) anterior palatine nerve; (18) greater palatine foramen.

SELF—TEST

Write in the names of the nerves on the lines provided below.

1. _____   10. _____
2. _____   11. _____
3. _____   12. _____
4. _____   13. _____
5. _____   14. _____
6. _____   15. _____
7. _____   16. _____
8. _____   17. _____
9. _____   18. _____

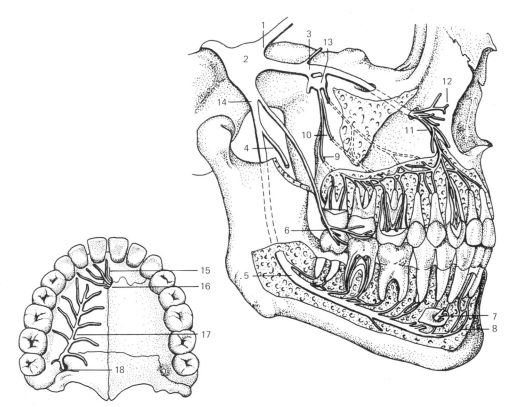

In Chapter 1 on pages 47–49 you learned that blood is a highly complex fluid with many unique functions; and although the blood is liquid, it is sometimes classed as a tissue. You also learned that nearly one-half of the blood is made up of solid particles, which include blood cells and blood platelets suspended in fluid (plasma).

The blood has three main functions: transportation, protection, and regulation. It transports the red blood cells that carry oxygen from the lungs to the body tissues, and carbon dioxide from the tissues to the lungs. It carries food to the tissues and removes waste. The white blood cells protect our bodies by fighting disease. The blood's regulatory functions are to control body temperature, carry hormones to all parts of the body, and maintain water content of all tissues. These functions are carried out by the exchange of blood through arteries, arterioles, and capillaries, and by its return, via the venules and veins, to be recirculated again.

The average adult has approximtely 5 to 6 quarts of blood; the circulatory system carries this entire quantity on one complete circuit through the body every minute. In the course of 24 hours, approximately 7,200 quarts of blood will pass through the heart.

Arteries

The blood enters the head by way of the *common carotid artery*, which then branches to become the internal and external carotid arteries. The names of the main branches of the external carotid artery that the dental student should be familiar with are as follows.

1. Infraorbital
2. Inferior alveolar
3. Facial
4. Lingual
5. Maxillary

Veins

Although it is important to be aware of the arterial blood supply from the heart to the head and neck, it is even more important for the dentist or for the auxiliary administering local anesthesia to know where the veins are located in relation to the nerves. Veins, unlike arteries, carry the blood to the heart; and also, unlike arteries, they may be more easily entered. However, injection directly into a vein may be toxic. Therefore, those administering local anesthesia must be careful when making an injection to aspirate prior to injecting. Then, if necessary, the needle can be repositioned to avoid any adverse reaction.

Venous blood from the head and neck drains into the internal jugular vein, which descends beside the internal carotid artery and then, lower down, continues beside the common carotid artery to empty into the superior vena cava.

Some of the veins that are important to the dental auxiliary are noted below.

1. *Facial vein*: This vein begins at the medial angle of the eye and then descends behind the facial artery, usually emptying into the internal jugular vein.
2. *Maxillary vein*: This vein accompanies the maxillary artery.
3. *Pterygoid venous plexus*: This network of many interlacing veins is between the temporal and the lateral pterygoid muscles. It joins with the facial vein. This rich network of veins must be avoided when injecting into this area.

NEW WORD

Aspirate: To draw out by suction. In the administering of local anesthesia, it means to draw back on the plunger of the syringe to determine if the needle is in a blood vessel. If it is, blood will be drawn back into the barrel of the syringe or into the cartridge, depending on the type of syringe being used.

It is helpful to remember that arteries often have the same name as the nerves, and in many instances the artery occupies the same canal.

Study the information and illustration below and on page 114 and then take the Self-Test on the page that follows.

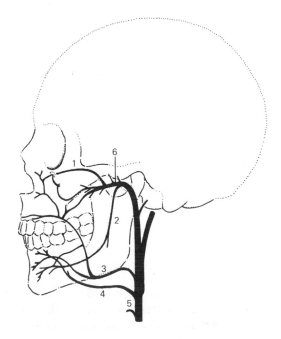

The main branches and some of the subbranches of the external carotid artery. (1) Infraorbital; (2) inferior alveolar; (3) facial; (4) lingual; (5) external carotid; (6) maxillary.

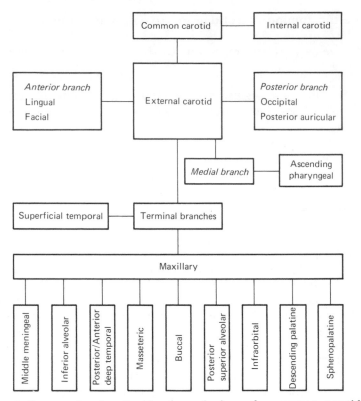

A diagram showing the blood supply from the common carotid artery to the external carotid artery and its branches.

SELF—TEST

Write in the names of the arteries shown on page 114 on the lines provided below.

1. _____

2. _____

3. _____

4. _____

5. _____

6. _____

The Lymphatic System of the Head and Neck

The lymphatic system is a part of the circulatory system. It is essentially a drainage system to carry off excess tissue fluid and waste. The lymph capillaries are the system's drainpipes. The fluid and waste thus disposed of are known as *lymph*. The lymph nodes within the system act as filtering stations and serve to retard the spread of infection. They manufacture lymphocytes and produce antibodies. The lymph capillaries join to form larger and larger lymphatic vessels comparable to veins. Eventually these vessels converge into two main channels. One channel is the right lymphatic duct, a short 7/16 inch (12 mm) tube that receives lymph from the right side of the head, neck, thorax, and the upper right extremities. The second is a 16 inch (40 cm) tube called the *thoracic duct*; this tube drains all parts of the body except those above the diaphragm on the right side. The thoracic duct extends upward through the diaphragm along the back wall of the thorax and into the root of the neck on the left side to eventually empty into a large vein. However, before the lymph reaches the vein, it must pass through a series of filters called *lymph nodes*, which filter the lymph to remove foreign particles. These lymph nodes are small rounded masses ranging from the size of a pin head to the size of an almond. They are massed in groups similar to bunches of grapes.

The tonsils are composed of lymphatic tissue and so are considered part of the lymphatic system. At times, in their attempt to protect the human body from infection, they will become greatly enlarged. The entire group of tonsils—palatine, pharyngeal, and lingual—is known as *Waldeyer's ring*.

The main lymph nodes are in the neck, axillae (armpit), and the groin. See the illustration below for the location of those in the head and neck that are important to the dental auxiliary.

Study the location of the lymph nodes in this illustration, then take the Self-Test on the following page.

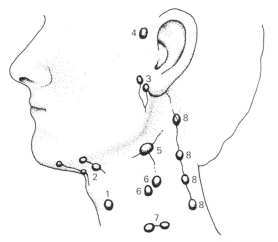

The lymph nodes of the head and neck. (1) Pretracheal; (2) submental, between the chin and the hyoid bone; (3) parotid; (4) preauricular; (5) subdigastric (master node); (6) medial (deep) cervical; (7) Supraclavicular; (8) posterior cervical chain.

SELF—TEST

Write in the names of the lymph nodes on the lines provided below.

1. _____

2. _____

3. _____

4. _____

5. _____

6. _____

7. _____

8. _____

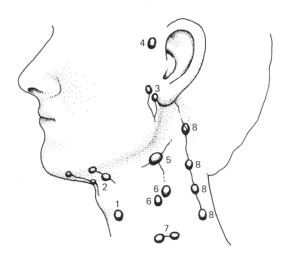

118

Dental
Histopathology

THE STAGES OF TOOTH DEVELOPMENT

Man is blessed with two sets of teeth: the first or *deciduous* teeth, and the second set or the *permanent* teeth. These sets of teeth were bestowed upon man to facilitate the mastication of food for the body's use, to enhance the esthetic appearance of the face, and to aid in speech. The study of the origin of the teeth, on through their various stages of development, is fascinating, for teeth are very complex. However, only a brief discussion of the developmental stages and the histopathology of the tissues involved will be offered in this text.

Unlike the bones of the skeleton that grow and calcify, or the organs of the various body systems that must grow and develop, the teeth must not only grow and calcify, but they must also erupt in order to perform their functions. All these stages occur in an orderly sequence. Should anything interfere with this sequence, an anomaly would develop (see below).

Initiation

The first phase of tooth development is initiation (bud stage). This begins in utero when the fetus is in the fifth or sixth week. At this time there will appear, in the primitive oral cavity, a thickening of the surface (oral) epithelium, forming a band along what will eventually become the alveolar ridges of the maxillae and the mandible. This epithelial band, called the *dental lamina*, contains cells capable of initiating the growth of the 20

119

deciduous teeth and the 32 permanent teeth. At certain points on the dental lamina small downgrowths will appear at different times, each representing the tooth bud of a deciduous tooth. After completing its functions involving the deciduous teeth, the dental lamina resorbs, except for the part supplying the succeeding permanent teeth and the posterior extensions that will initiate the nonsuccedaneous permanent molars.

Nature's plan during this stage does not always follow the prescribed pattern, and anomalies do occur. One such anomaly could be *partial anodontia*, which means the absence of one tooth; or there could be *complete anodontia*, meaning the absence of all teeth. Anodontia appears to be a hereditary trait and most frequently seems to involve the permanent lateral incisors, the third molars, and the lower second premolars. *Supranumerary* (extra) teeth may also develop when abnormal initiation occurs. Generally, the most common sites for supernumerary teeth to develop are in the area of the maxillary central incisors and in the area distal to the molars.

Proliferation

The second phase of tooth development is proliferation (rapid reproduction), which includes the bud and early cap stages. During this phase, the cells from the deepest layer of the dental lamina begin to multiply rapidly, increasing in size and changing shape. This action takes place in each jaw, resulting in the appearance of small buds (resembling caps) that dip down into the underlying mesoderm. The first deciduous tooth buds to appear are in the anterior mandibular region. The other tooth buds follow at different times and will correspond to the sites of the remaining deciduous teeth. There are 20 in all. The tooth buds of the 20 permanent succedaneous teeth (in place of) appear about the fourth or fifth month in utero. These buds appear from a lingual extension of the dental lamina that gave rise to the deciduous tooth buds. However, the tooth buds of the nonsuccedaneous permanent molars will develop directly from the dental limina as it extends toward the posterior of the mouth. The tooth buds of the nonsuccedaneous permanent molars develop at various times—from the fourth month of fetal life for the first permanent molar, to the fourth or fifth year of life for the third permanent molar.

Tooth Bud. The tooth bud consists of *three parts*, all of which have a particular part to play in the formation of the entire tooth and the periodontium.

Dental Organ. The first part of the tooth bud is the dental organ, sometimes called the *enamel organ*. It is derived from the ectodermal layer and gives rise to the enamel that will in time cover the entire crown of the tooth.

Dental Papilla. The second part, the dental papilla, is derived from the underlying mesodermal layer. It forms within the invagination of the dental organ and is responsible for the dentin, which forms the bulk of the tooth, and for the pulp that contains the tooth's vital parts.

Dental Sac. The third part, the dental sac, is also derived from the under-lying mesodermal layer, and it will eventually surround the dental organ and the dental papilla. It is responsible for the periodontal ligaments that hold the tooth in the alveolus (socket), as well as for the cementum and for the alveolar bone that serves as a place of attachment for the periodontal ligaments.

At first, the dental organ will appear as a simple rounded body dropping down from the dental lamina. Soon, however, a change may be noted as the dental organ lengthens into a short, slender cord of epithelial cells extending down into the embryonic connective tissue (mesoderm). Mitotic activity is evident at this time in both the epithelial tissue of the dental organ and in the underlying connective tissue. As the cells of the dental organ continue to proliferate, a shallow invagination on the inferior surface will form, giving it the appearance of a cap. Further proliferation results in deepening the invagi-nation of the dental organ, which now takes on the shape of a bell. The epithelial cells lining the invagination now form four separate layers that will influence the further development of the tooth. These four layers are described below.

1. *Outer dental epithelium*: The outer dental epithelium (external layer) lines the highest convexity of the invaginated dental organ and appears to serve, for a time, as a source of nutrients for the inner dental epithelium.
2. *Inner dental epithelium*: This layer lines the concavity of the dental organ and will ultimately differentiate into enamel-forming cells called *ameloblasts*.
3. *Stellate reticulum*: Between the outer dental epithelium and the inner dental epithelium is the third layer, the stellate reticulum. This layer is composed of cells that are separated by wide intercellular spaces filled with a cushioning fluid that seems to give support and protection to the developing tooth germ.
4. *Stratum intermedium*: Between the inner dental epithelium and the stellate reticulum is the fourth layer, the stratum intermedium. This layer appears to have some influence on the production of enamel.

Differentiation

The third phase in the formation of a tooth is differentiation, which occurs during the late cap stage and the early bell stage. The cells now prac-tically cease to proliferate and prepare to perform their assigned functions. During this stage the dental lamina that has furnished attachment to the oral epithelium for the dental organ will begin to disintegrate. The connective tissue cells of the dental papilla that face the inner dental epithelium begin to differentiate and assume a columnar form. They are now dentin-forming cells, the *odontoblasts*. Soon after this occurs, the cells of the inner epithelium differentiate into ameloblasts. These two layers of cells, one of ectodermal origin and the other of mesodermal origin, are separated by a thin membrane that is the future site of the dentino-enamel junction (where dentin and enamel meet).

The cells' individual roles have now been established, and many things are occurring. The connective tissue around the inferior part of the dental papilla is beginning to appear fibrous. This is the beginning of the dental sac that will eventually enclose the entire dental organ, severing its connection with the surface. The connective tissue cells within the dental sac, during this phase, will be differentiating into *cementoblasts*, which will form cementum to envelop the root of the tooth; *fibroblasts*, which will form the periodontal ligaments; and *osteoblasts*, which will play a part in forming the alveolar bone surrounding the tooth. During the final stages of differentiation, the secondary lamina for the succeeding permanent tooth has appeared to the lingual of the developing primary tooth, and the dental organ of the permanent tooth is proceeding to develop in the same manner as did that of the deciduous tooth.

Hertwig's Sheath. When the enamel and dentin of the tooth crown are complete, the inner and outer layers of epithelium fuse, forming Hertwig's sheath. This sheath is responsible for root and dentin formation. It takes the form of one or more epithelial tubes, depending on the number of roots involved, such as three for the maxillary molars and two for the mandibular, etc. After the functions of Hertwig's sheath are completed, it is resorbed. However, remnants remain in the periodontal ligament near the root surface and are known as *epithelial rests*. At times, the remains of Hertwig's sheath are stimulated to differentiate into ameloblasts. Anomalies will then occur, usually at the bifurcation or trifurcation of molar roots. These anomalies are called *enamel pearls*.

Anomalies. During the final stage of differentiation (morphodifferentiation), other anomalies occur as the cells are assuming their individual roles.

Fusion. One such anomaly is the joining of tooth germs (buds), usually resulting in a large crown with two roots, or in one grooved root with two canals.

Gemination. Gemination occurs when a single tooth germ separates to form two crowns on a single root.

Dens in Dente. Dens in dente is sometimes called "tooth within a tooth," because this is the way the anomaly appears in a radiograph (x-ray). It results when the epithelial layers within the dental organ invaginate *into* the underlying dental papilla, forming a small cavity that contains a hard structure resembling a tooth. This usually involves the maxillary lateral incisor. A tooth such as this usually has a very uncertain future.

1. Initiation:
    Bud stage

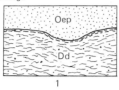

2. Proliferation:
    Bud and
    early cap stage

3. Differentiation:
    Late cap stage and
    early bell stage

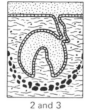

4. Apposition:
    Late bell stage
    and
    early calcification

5. Calcification:

6. Eruption:

7. Attrition:

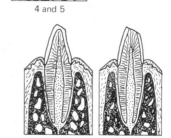

The seven phases of tooth development.

Apposition

Apposition is the fourth phase of tooth development, and it is during this phase that a rhythmic laying down of organic substance, water, and mineral salts results in the enamel matrix. One anomaly that can be caused by a disease such as measles is *enamel hypoplasia* (reduced enamel); all teeth developing at this time will be affected.

Calcification

During calcification, the fifth phase, almost all of the organic substance becomes increasingly impregnated with mineral salts.

Eruption

During eruption, the sixth phase, the tooth moves toward and enters the oral cavity. This is known as *active* eruption.

Passive eruption occurs in four stages throughout a person's lifetime. In stages I and II the anatomical crown is larger than the clinical crown; in stage III the two crowns are equal; in stage IV the clinical crown is larger due to recession.

Attrition

The seventh and final phase is the normal wearing away of the incisal and occlusal surfaces of the teeth through mastication.

Although the development of a tooth has been given in phases, one must remember that all these phases overlap and act interchangeably, as do all phases of embryological development.

SELF–TEST

1. What are the names for the first and the second sets of teeth? _____

_____

2. Name three functions of our teeth.
   (a) _____
   (b) _____
   (c) _____
3. Name the seven phases of tooth development, and briefly describe each.

   (a) _____

   (b) _____

   (c) _____

   (d) _____

   (e) _____

   (f) _____

   (g) _____
4. At what period of time, in utero, do the first teeth begin to develop?

_____

5. How many teeth are there in the first dentition? Second? _____

6. What does *succedaneous* mean? _____

7. Define *anodontia*. What teeth are most apt to be involved? _____

8. Define *supernumerary*. What areas are most apt to be involved? _____
_____

9. Define *proliferation*. _____

10. Do the secondary teeth develop to the lingual or the distal of the first teeth? _____

11. Do the first, second, and third molars develop from an extension of the epithelial cells that formed the first teeth, or do they develop directly from the oral epithelium? _____

12. What is another name for the dental organ? _____

13. Name the three parts of the tooth bud and tell what parts of the tooth develop from each.

    (a) _____

    (b) _____

    (c) _____

14. Which cells form enamel? Dentin? _____

15. Hertwig's sheath is responsible for what part of the tooth? _____

16. Briefly define *fusion, gemination, dens in dente*. _____
_____
_____

17. What does the term *enamel hypoplasia* mean? What is its cause, and during what stage of tooth development does it occur? _____
_____

THE TOOTH TISSUES

Enamel

Enamel, dentin, cementum, and the pulp are the tooth tissues. Enamel is the tissue that covers the entire anatomical crown of the tooth. It is the hardest tissue in the body. This hardness is derived from inorganic material, primarily calcium phosphate, which makes up 97% of this tissue. Nature has arranged enamel in such a way that the parts of the tooth receiving the most wear from mastication also have the thickest layer of enamel, a layer that usually measures from 2 mm to 2.6 mm depending on its location. For all its hardness, enamel is brittle and will fracture. It is also susceptible to acid-forming bacteria found in the oral cavity, and it can be worn down on the incisal and occlusal surfaces (biting surfaces) through mastication. Once destroyed through trauma, bacterial invasion, or attrition, enamel is incapable of repair because its formative organ (dental organ) has been lost through the process of eruption and mastication. Originally the epithelial remains of the dental organ covered the crown of the newly erupted tooth, protecting it for a time as the tooth erupted. This layer of epithelial cells is known as the *enamel cuticle* (Nasmyth's membrane). However, it is soon worn away from the exposed surfaces.

Form. The basement membrane that separates the ameloblasts from the odontoblasts during the differentiation phase of development forms the pattern for the occlusal or incisal part of the crown of all teeth. A longitudinal section will show this juntion to be scalloped. This pattern is due to convex projections of enamel fitting snugly into concavities in the dentin, locking the cap of enamel securely to the dentin. During the beginning stages (as mentioned previously), activity begins at this basement membrane, with the inner enamel epithelium influencing the underlying connective tissue cells to produce odontoblasts. This activity is an essential stimulus to the production of dentin, which begins in the cuspal areas of the future dentino-enamel junction, and is also an essential activity prior to the production of the enamel matrix, which is first laid down in a thin layer along the basement membrane after the first dentin has been deposited. The enamel matrix then progresses outwardly to eventually complete the pattern for a given tooth. Mineralization is taking place at the same time as the matrix is being formed, with the incisal and occlusal surfaces completed first.

Structure. In general, the enamel of a tooth is composed of millions of rods (or prisms) with anywhere from 8,000,000 rods in an incisor to 12,000,000 rods in a molar. These rods extend from the dentino-enamel junction to the surface in a wavelike manner. The direction they take depends on the crown's form. Near the dentino-enamel junction, these rods assume a twisted and curved pattern extending toward the cusps of the posterior teeth. On the incisors the rods are straight. This twisted and curved enamel is extremely hard and is called *gnarled enamel*. Its form is a factor to be considered in cavity preparation. Each enamel rod is encased in a rod sheath that is slightly less inorganic than the rod, and both rod and sheath are held together by a minute amount of interrod substance that is comparatively softer. It has been noted that when a split occurs in enamel, it is along the interrod substance, making this also a factor in cavity preparation.

Stripes of Retzius. Microscopic examination shows many structures within enamel. One such structure is the stripes of Retzius. These brownish areas are formed by the laying down of small particles of poorly calcified enamel in incremental layers, one above the other, similar to growth rings in trees.

Enamel Lamellae. During the formative period, tears or cracks occur in the surface of the enamel. These areas usually extend toward or into the dentin; they are poorly calcified and logically serve as an easy entry for bacteria.

Enamel Tufts. Enamel tufts are poorly calcified enamel that resemble small treelike objects erupting at intervals from the dentino-enamel junction. They extend into the enamel for some distance, and may account for the pattern taken by dental caries as it approaches the dentin.

Enamel Spindles. Enamel spindlelike processes are continuations of the odontoblastic processes within the dentinal tubules (spaces in dentin). They were probably formed prior to mineralization of the enamel and thus were entrapped. These extensions may account for apparent sensitivity at the dentino-enamel junction when approached during cavity preparation.

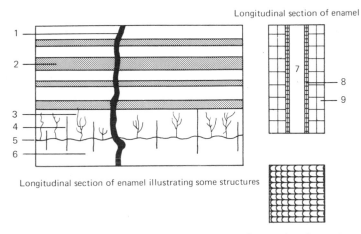

Longitudinal section of enamel illustrating some structures. (1) Lamellae; (2) stripes of Retzius; (3) enamel tufts; (4) enamel spindles; (5) dentino-enamel junction; (6) dentin; (7) rod; (8) sheath; (9) interrod substance.

SELF—TEST

1. Name the four tooth tissues. _____

_____

2. Which tissue covers the entire anatomical crown of a tooth? _____

3. What percentage of this tissue is inorganic? _____

4. Is it the hardest tissue in the body? _____

5. Where, on the tooth, is this tissue thickest? Why? _____

6. Name three things that might destroy this tissue. _____

_____

7. Why can't this tissue be self-repairing? _____

8. What is Nasmyth's membrane? Explain. _____

_____

9. Where does this tissue first form? _____

10. In what direction does this tissue form after the first layer is laid down?

_____

11. What is this tissue composed of? Give the structure. _____

_____

12. What is the twisted tissue called? Is is harder than other parts of the same tissue? _____

_____

13. Briefly describe "stripes of Retzius." _____

14. Cracks and tears occur in the surface of this tissue and appear to be ideal spots for bacterial invasion. What are they called? _____

15. Describe and name the tufts found along the dentino-enamel junction.

16. Do odontoblastic processes extend past the dentino-enamel junction into this tissue? If so, what are they called? _____

_____

Dentin

Dentin is the calcified tissue that lies under the enamel in the crown of the tooth and under the cementum in the root. It forms the bulk of the tooth, giving it elasticity, strength, and form. It is 70% inorganic, making it harder than cementum and bone but not so hard as enamel. It is slightly brownish yellow in color and completely devoid of blood vessels and cells.

Form. The odontoblasts (dentin-forming cells) form on the pulpal side of the basement membrane; and as a layer of dentin is laid down, the odonto-blasts draw away by elongation from this membrane while the pulp recedes, so that they are always located on the pulpal surface. As the odontoblasts recede from the basement membrane, they leave behind extensions embedded in the matrix. These extensions are called *processes*. When the dentin has been completed, the odontoblasts remain on the surface of the pulp and do not function unless stimulated to produce secondary dentin.

Structure. Dentin is composed of matrix, slightly curved tubules with one odontoblastic process (fiber) in each tubule. The dentin is laid down in increments in much the same manner as enamel, showing a similar growth pattern.

Matrix. The foundation of dentin is the dentinal matrix, a solid but elastic substance consisting of minute fibrils held together by a cementing substance containing calcium salts. Perforating this matrix are innumerable minute canals called *dentinal tubules*.

Tubules. The dentinal tubules, or channels, extend from the dentino-enamel junction to the pulp chamber in the crown and to the pulp canals in the roots. Within each of these tubules is a soft elastic fiber called the *dental fiber*, which is the remains of the odontoblastic process.

Fibers. The dentinal fibers, also called *Tome's fibers*, are extensions of the odontoblasts that lie next to the dentin on the inner periphery of the pulp. These dentinal fibers branch out at the dentino-enamel junction; and irritations during cavity preparation possibly are transmitted through them to the many nerve endings in the pulp, accounting for sensitivity in that area.

Interglobular Dentin. Interglobular dentin refers to the undercalcified areas found primarily in the dentin lying next to the dentino-enamel junction. They are thought to represent imperfect calcifications, or fusion of the matrix during the time the tooth was forming.

Tome's Granular Layer. Tome's granular layer is the irregular outer layer of noncalcified dentin lying next to the cementum. It is possibly caused by a disturbance during calcification of this layer of dentin.

Predentin. Predentin is the newest layer of noncalcified dentin that lies closest to the pulp. It is found in young teeth.

Korff's Fibers. Korff's fibers are thick bundles of fibers that lie between the odontoblasts lining the inner periphery of the pulp. They extend into the noncalcified predentin and appear to have some function in matrix production.

Secondary Dentin. Secondary dentin is modified dentin found in older teeth. This type of dentin forms on the inner pulpal wall. It forms throughout the life of the tooth as long as the pulp is intact. It may form as a reaction to trauma, dental caries, or other stimuli. Its function is to protect the pulp. It is sometimes referred to as reparative dentin.

Sclerotic Dentin. Sclerotic dentin is modified dentin, most often seen in the elderly. It appears also to be a defensive reaction to attrition and gingival recession where dentin is exposed to wear, stain, etc.

Anomaly. *Dentinogenesis imperfecta* (opalescent dentin) is a hereditary disturbance. Both deciduous and permanent teeth are affected. The teeth appear gray. Attrition is rapid, and carious lesions are not uncommon. In a modification of dentinogenesis imperfecta, the roots of the teeth fail to form and the pulp chamber is wide. These teeth are called *shell teeth*. The diagrammatic illustrations on the next page show a portion of the structure of tooth dentin and relation of dentin to pulp and enamel.

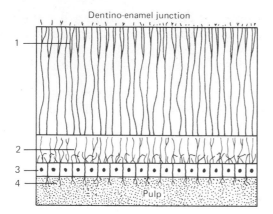

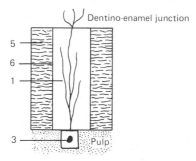

Structural parts of dentin. (1) Dentinal fibers; (2) predentin; (3) odontoblasts; (4) Korff's fibers; (5) matrix; (6) tubule.

SELF—TEST

1. Is dentin found in both the crown and the root of the tooth? _____

2. What percentage of inorganic matter does it contain? _____

3. On which side of the basement membrane do the odontoblasts form?
_____

4. Do the odontoblasts extend toward the pulp or from the pulp as dentin
   is laid down? _____

5. When dentin is completed, what happens to the odontoblast? _____

6. Dentin is composed of _____

7. What is another name for dentinal fibers? _____

8. What is predentin, and where is it found? _____

9. What appears to be the function of Korff's fibers, and where are they
   located? _____

_____

10. Define *secondary dentin*; *sclerotic dentin*. _____

_____

11. Is dentinogenesis imperfecta thought to be hereditary? _____

12. What is the appearance of the teeth when dentinogenesis imperfecta is present? _____

The Pulp

The pulp of the tooth might be compared to the vital organs of the body, for it is the vital part of the tooth. However, when the vital organs of the body die, the body dies; but when the pulp dies, the pulp chamber and the canal, or canals, can be filled with gutta percha (a latex material from Malaysian trees) and/or silver points, and the tooth is again a functional organ. This treatment is called *endodontics*.

Structure. The pulp is a noncalcified structure composed of blood vessels, nerves, lymphatic vessels, intercellular substance, connective tissue cells, and Korff's fibers. It is the remains of the dental papilla that formed the dentin during the embryological phase of tooth development. It occupies a cavity in the center of the dentin. This cavity consists of the pulp chamber, pulpal horns, and the pulp canal or canals. Many times tiny lateral branches can be seen extending from the pulp canal; and in many teeth, accessory canals are found. In young persons the pulp canals are wide with a large opening at their apices; however, as a person ages, the pulp canals become narrower due to the continuous deposition of secondary dentin. At the apex of each root is a foramen that allows the nerves, blood vessels, and lymph to enter through the pulp canal into the pulp chamber.

Functions. The pulp has numerous functions: one of its most important is *formative*, or the ability to form secondary dentin. Another is *sensation*, for the pulp responds to thermal, chemical, or traumatic irritation with pain. This pain response can cause "referred" pain to any point on the side affected, due to the location of the branches of the trigeminal nerve. A dentist will check all teeth to the midline to determine the specific cause of pain. A third function is *nutritive*, as the pulp nourishes the dentin via the odontoblastic processes. The last but not least is the *defensive* reaction of the pulp. When the pulp is in danger, an inflammatory response occurs and secondary (reparative) dentin is laid down in an attempt to protect the pulp. Occasionally this response is also the cause of pulpal death when excessive pressure from the fluid content of inflammation is forced into the bone surrounding the apex, and endodontic treatment is necessary to save the tooth from extraction.

Cells of the Pulp

1. *Odontoblast*: A connective tissue cell that forms dentin.
2. *Histeocyte*: Part of the pulp's defense system. It responds to inflammation by ingesting and destroying waste and harmful bacteria. This process is called *phagocytosis*.
3. *Fibroblast*: An immature fiber-producing cell capable of differentiating into a chondroblast, collagenoblast, or osteoblast.

Diseases. Some common diseases of the pulp are described below.

Pulpitis (toothache). Acute pulpitis can be caused by many things, such as thermal excesses, trauma, chemicals, or bacterial invasion—any of which can trigger severe pain. Some pulpitis is chronic and has a milder but longer pain response. Untreated, either condition may lead to pulpal death.

Granuloma. A dental granuloma is an apical extension of pulpal inflammation. It will appear as an area of radiolucency of varying width in a radiograph due to the replacement of alveolar bone and periodontal ligament with granulation tissue.

Cyst. A radicular cyst is a cavity lined with epithelium that often results from a deep carious lesion or restoration. It appears radiolucent in a radiograph, and when removed, it is saclike in appearance. It is filled with either necrotic debris or fluid.

Pulp stones. Pulp stones (denticles) are nonpathologic calcifications of different types; they may interfere with instrumentation during endodontic treatment. Their cause is not known. They may at times be seen in radiographs as a radiopaque area within the pulp.

NEW WORDS

Chondroblast (kon′-dro-blast): An immature cartilage-producing cell.

Collagenoblast (kol-laj′-e-no-blast″): An immature collagen-producing cell.

Endodontics (en″-do-don′-tiks): The branch of dentistry concerned with the etiology, prevention, diagnosis, and treatment of conditions that affect the dental pulp and the periapical tissues.

Etiology (e″-te-ol′-o-je): The science dealing with causes of disease.

Gutta percha (gut″-ta pur′-cha): A rubberlike substance of tropical plant origin; a shapeless solid, insoluble in water, partly soluble in hot alcohol, almost completely soluble in chloroform. It comes from Malaysian trees.

Periapical (per′-e-a″-pi-cal): Tissues surrounding the apex of a tooth.

Radiolucent (ra″-de-o-lu′-sent): Permitting the passage of radiant energy such as Xrays, yet offering some resistance to it, the representative areas appearing dark on the exposed film.

Radiopaque (ra″-de-o-pāk): Stopping the passage of radiant energy. The representative areas appearing white or in shades of grey, depending on the density of the tissues involved.

SELF—TEST

1. When the pulp dies, can the tooth still be saved? If so, how? _____

_____

2. Where is the pulp located in relation to the dentin? _____

3. Are the pulp canals and the openings at the apex of a tooth in a young person larger or smaller? _____

4. Name four functions of the pulp. _____

_____

5. Name the three cells of the pulp. _____

6. What is pulpitis? _____

7. What is the difference between a granuloma and a cyst? _____

8. Are pulp stones pathologic? How do they appear in radiographs? _____

_____

9. Define *radiopaque*. _____

10. Define *radiolucency*. _____

Cementum

Cementum is one of the most important of the tooth tissues. If enamel and dentin are destroyed, the tooth can still be made functional through restorative dentistry. If the pulp of the tooth dies, the tooth can still be made functional through endodontics. But, if the entire cementum layer is lost, so is the tooth. This very important tissue protects the root dentin of our teeth from resorption, and it also furnishes attachment for the periodontal fibers, thus aiding in the retention of the tooth in the socket. Another function of the cementum is to compensate for occlusal wear by continually adding a layer of cementum to the apical area of the root.

The arrangement of cementum at the cemento-enamel junction varies. At times the thin layers of cementum and enamel just meet at the cemento-enamel junction. At other times they do not quite meet, leaving a small area of dentin exposed, which appears to result in some senitivity in that area. Therefore, great caution should be observed during an oral prophylaxsis. The most frequent, or most common, arrangement, however, is the slight overlapping of the enamel by the cementum at the cemento-enamel junction.

Structure. Cementum is composed of matrix, cementoblasts, cementocytes, lacunae, canaliculi, embedded fibers, and acellular cementum.

Matrix. The matrix of the cementum consists of fibrous tissue held together by a calcified cementing substance. It is almost identical to the matrix of bone. It is approximately 50% inorganic.

Lacunae. Lacunae (lah-ku'-nah) are minute cavities, or spaces, in cellular cementum. They are occupied by cementocytes that have become entrapped during mineralization.

Cementocytes. Cementocytes frequently have long processes radiating from the cell body toward the periodontal surface of the cementum. They are found in the lacunae of cellular cementum.

Canaliculi. Canaliculi are small canals or channels in cellular cementum that branch out from the lacunae, allowing the long processes of the entrapped cementocytes to extend toward their source of nutrition—the periodontal ligament.

Acellular Cementum. Acellular cementum is cementum without cells. When root dentin begins to form, cells from the inner border of the dental sac arrange themselves on the outer surface of the dentin and begin depositing cementum, layer upon layer. These cells then remain on the surface of the root dentin in much the same manner as the dentin-forming cells remain on the inner periphery of the pulp. This acellular cementum is found around all root surfaces; however, it is occasionally absent in the most apical portion.

Cellular Cementum. Cellular cementum, or cementum with cells, generally is formed over the apical area of the root, and over the acellular cementum if it is present. If the acellular cementum is absent in that area, the cellular cementum forms directly over the dentin.

Cementoid Tissue. Cementum is deposited in layers in much the same manner as enamel and dentin. The first layer is an uncalcified cementoid tissue that becomes calcified as layer after layer of this thin uncalcified tissue is deposited. Fibers from the periodontal ligament will become securely embedded in this cementoid tissue and in the underlying cementum.

Sharpey's Fibers. Sharpey's fibers are connective tissue fibers from the periodontal ligament that pass between the cementoblasts that line the outer periphery of the root and into the softer cementoid tissue that lines the root of the tooth. They then extend into the cementum where they are embedded, furnishing attachment of the tooth to the surrounding bone.

Anomaly. *Hypercementosis* is not necessarily a pathological condition. It is just an abnormal thickening of the cementum. However, at times when there has been extensive occlusal stress, there may be such an excess of cementum around the apex of the tooth that it will be firmly attached to the bone of the alveolus. This condition is called *ankylosis*. An ankylosed tooth needing extraction would probably indicate that some of the alveolar bone would also have to be removed.

SELF—TEST

1. Name three functions of the cementum. ⸻

2. Name three possible arrangements of cementum at the cemento-enamel junction. ⸻

3. What is cementum composed of? ⸻

4. What percentage of inorganic material is found in cementum? ⸻

5. Is cementum comparable to bone in structure and hardness? ⸻

6. Define *lacunae*; *canaliculi*. ⸻

7. Is the outer cementum next to the periodontal ligament less calcified than the inner layer? What is this layer called? ⸻

8. What are Sharpey's fibers? ⸻

9. Explain *hypercementosis*. ⸻

10. What is the meaning of ankylosis? ⸻

THE SUPPORTING TISSUES

Periodontal Ligament

The periodontal ligament is noncalcified and of connective tissue origin. It is a product of the dental sac. Sharpey's fibers, part of this very important tissue, are embedded deeply, on one side, into the bone of the alveolus (tooth socket), and on the other side, into the cementum that surrounds the roots of the tooth, suspending the tooth in the socket. Because of this relationship, cementum is not only a tooth tissue but is a supporting tissue as well. The periodontal ligament is just another of nature's ingenuous devices to keep us functioning, for without this versatile suspensory ligament, the teeth would be lost, and frequently are, when these fibers have been weakened or destroyed through neglect, trauma, irritation, or poor diet.

Structure. The periodontal ligaments are arranged in bundles forming six groups. These six groups are called the *principal fibers* (see description on p. 136). They extend from the cementum to the gingiva and from the cementum to the alveolus, preventing the tooth from being rotated or jammed down into the socket during mastication. Between the bundles of ligaments are blood vessels, nerves, other strategically placed fibers, and cells. The cells are the osteoblasts, cementoblasts, osteoclasts, fibroblasts and histiocytes. The osteoblasts, which build the wall of the alveolus, remain against the bone and between the principal fibers where bone is forming. The cementoblasts lie along the root of the tooth between the ligaments and have the same relationship to cementum as the osteoblasts have to bone. The osteoclasts are destroyers of hard tissue whenever this is necessary; they then disappear until again needed. The fibroblasts lie between the fibers, maintaining the integrity of the principal fibers. The histiocytes are phagocytic cells (defense cells) located strategically, ready to perform when inflammation is present.

Principal Fibers. The principal fibers of the periodonal ligament are composed of six groups that are named according to their location. These fibers are listed below:

Free Gingival. The free gingival fibers pass from the cementum into the free and attached gingiva holding the gingiva firmly to the tooth surface.

Transeptal. The transeptal fibers are just apical to the free gingival fibers. These fibers help maintain the teeth in their proper relationship. They extend from the cementum of one tooth to the cementum of the adjacent tooth.

Alveolar Crest. The alveolar crest fibers are embedded on one side in the cementum of the tooth root at the cervix, and on the other side in the alveolar crest. They surround the tooth and resist horizontal movement.

Horizontal. The horizontal fibers are apical to the alveolar crest fibers and are embedded in the cementum of the tooth root and in the bone of the alveolus. They lie in a horizontal position all around the tooth root and resist horizontal pressures that are applied to the crown.

Oblique. The oblique fibers are apical to the horizontal fibers and are attached to the cementum and bone in an oblique direction, with the end that is attached to the bone more toward the crown than the end that is attached to the cementum. This arrangement prevents the apex from jamming against the bottom of the socket.

Apical. The apical fibers radiate around the apex of the tooth in a right angle to their attachment in the bone at the base of the alveolus, thus resisting forces that tend to remove the tooth from the socket. They also stabilize against forces tending to produce tilting.

Diseases. There are many diseases, or pathologies, of the periodontal ligament. Only a few will be briefly discussed in this text.

Periodontal Abscess. A parulis (pah-roo'-lis), or abscess, is a localized collection of pus in a cavity formed by the disintegration of tissue. It is a natural defense mechanism by means of which the body attempts to localize an infection. The periodontal abscess is, of course, associated with periodontal disease, and it frequently forms in deep periodontal pockets, an ideal place to incubate bacteria. It is usually like a small boil on the gingiva or alveolar mucosa. It is not painful but may rupture and discharge pus. It is generally treated by incision and drainage. Many times an antibiotic will be prescribed.

Gingivitis. There are many types of gingivitis, an inflammation of the gingivae, and each type has a different etiologic agent. Two of the most common types are described below.

Hyperplastic gingivitis: Hyperplastic gingivitis is common among those who must take the drug dilantin to control epileptic seizures. This condition is distinguished by an excessive overgrowth of gingival tissue, which at times is so extensive it must be removed surgically.
Hormonal gingivitis: Hormonal gingivitis is a type of gingivitis that occurs during various stages of a person's lifetime when the body is undergoing hormonal change. This condition is recognized by enlarged, red puffy gingivae that bleed easily; it is associated with a health history record indicating pregnancy or changes due to a particular age.

Periodontitis. At times if gingivitis is not corrected, periodontitis may be the end result. Calculus is usually present in great amounts; local factors such as overhangs on restorations and dental plaque cause a breakdown in the ligament and a detachment from the tooth (periodontal pocket), with ultimate destruction of the alveolar crest.

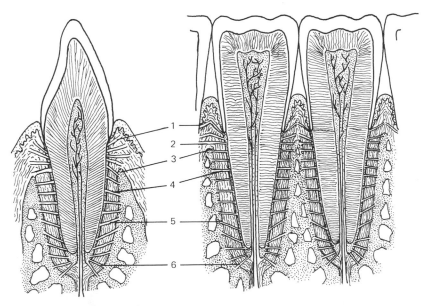

Parts of the principal fibers of the periodontal ligament. (1) Gingival; (2) transeptal; (3) alveolar crest; (4) horizontal; (5) oblique; (6) apical.

Although the dental auxiliary does not diagnose, he or she must be able to recognize certain conditions when performing preliminary intra-oral examinations.

The diagrammatic illustration on page 137 shows the location of the six principal fibers of the periodontal membrane.

Periodontosis. Periodontosis is a degenerative disease of the periodontal tissues. The collagen fibers of the periodontal ligament degenerate, and a deep pocket forms. The teeth will migrate, causing problems such as malocclusion and extrusion; supporting bone is lost; and the teeth become loose. This condtion is thought to be systemic. However, little is known concerning its origin.

SELF—TEST

1. The periodontal ligament is a product of what part of the dental germ?
   _____

2. Is it a tooth tissue or a supporting tissue? _____

3. Name the six groups of principal fibers of the periodontal ligament. _____
   _____

4. What cells are found in the periodontal ligament? _____

5. What is a parulis? _____

6. Define *hyperplastic gingivitis.* _____

7. What drug contributes to this condition? _____

8. Can a pregnant woman have gingivitis? _____

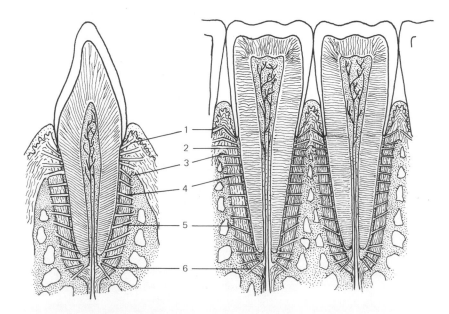

9. What is the difference between periodontitis and periodontosis? _____

Alveolar Bone

The alveolar process is a product of the embryonic dental sac, which also gives rise to the cementum and the periodontal ligament. About the second month in utero a groove forms that is open to the oral cavity. Within this groove are bony crypts, and within these crypts lie the tooth germs of the deciduous teeth. Gradually bony septa form between the tooth germs, and as the teeth erupt, the alveolar process develops around them. It appears that this growth is the driving force in tooth eruption.[2] Ultimately the alveolar process will rest upon, and become indistinguishable from, the bone of the maxillae and mandible that develop later. The periosteum that forms over the cortical plate (outer bony plate) of the alveolar process will also, in due time, become one with that covering the cortical plate of the maxillae and mandible.

Like the deciduous teeth, the permanent teeth lie in bony crypts; but unlike the deciduous teeth, the permanent teeth are almost entirely enclosed by bone, leaving only a small opening toward the oral cavity to allow the epithelial strand (dental lamina) to pass. As these teeth erupt, the bone over the occlusal or incisal edges will resorb, allowing the teeth to erupt into the oral cavity.

Composition. The alveolar bone is composed of an outer covering called a *cortical plate*, which is a thin, compact solid bone containing no empty spaces. Between this outer plate is cancellous bone containing many empty marrow spaces, giving it a spongy appearance. The calcified matrix within this cancelleous bone is arranged in trabeculae (trah-bek′-ū-laē) (bundles of fibers), which aid in the support of the alveolus during masticatory stress. These trabeculae are arranged in either a horizontal or vertical fashion, depending on their location.

The bone that lines the alveolus (socket) is thin and has many openings to allow the blood vessels, nerves, and lymphatics to reach and nourish the periodontal ligament. Sharpey's fibers from the periodontal ligament are embedded in this bone, aiding in the support of the teeth in their sockets. This normal attachment is called *gomphosis*. In a roentgenogram (Xray) this layer of alveolar bone appears as a white line that is somewhat thicker on the distal than the mesial, due to the mesial drift of all teeth. This thin line of bone is called the *lamina dura*.

[2]Issac Schour, *Oral Histology and Embryology*, 8th ed. (Philadelphia: Lea & Febinger, 1960), p. 199.

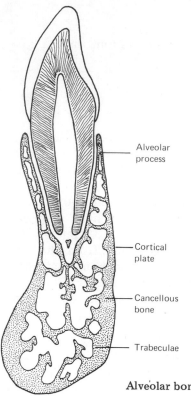

Alveolar process

Cortical plate

Cancellous bone

Trabeculae

Alveolar bone composition.

NEW WORDS

Crypt: A cavity.

Gomphosis: Normal attachment of the periodontal ligament to the cementum and the alveolus.

Roentgenogram: Xray.

SELF—TEST

1. Is the alveolar process a product of the same embryonic part of the dental germ (tooth bud), as is the periodontal ligament? _____

2. Does the alveolar process develop as the teeth erupt? _____

3. What is the periosteum? _____

4. What is the composition of alveolar bone? _____

5. Are Sharpey's fibers embedded in this bone? _____

6. Could the alveolar bone be considered a supporting tissue? _____

7. Define *gomphosis*. _____

8. What are trabeculae? _____

9. What is the lamina dura? _____

10. Locate the various parts of the alveolar bone on the drawing on page 141.

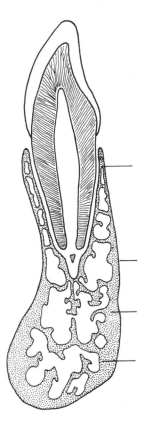

The Gingiva

The gingiva is, in most cases, a *keratinized* tissue that surrounds the teeth. Nature designed this tissue to protect the underlying soft tissues from trauma during the mastication of food. In appearance, when healthy, the attached gingiva is firm, and stippled somewhat like the stippling on an orange. The color of the gingiva will vary in certain ethnic groups, ranging from grayish pink to brown. Edematose, red, shiny, and smooth gingiva indicate inflammation is present. When teaching preventive care, the dental auxiliary must be able to distinguish between healthy and unhealthy gingiva. Also when scaling and polishing the teeth, the dental auxiliary must have a general knowledge of the gingiva and associated structures and tissues in order to prevent injury to the patient. In this section only a very brief description of those areas thought to be most important will be discussed.

Epithelial Attachment. During the eruption of the tooth, the epithelial layer covering the tip of the tooth fuses with the oral epithelium. The attached epithelium separates from the tooth to form a shallow sulcus (groove) as eruption continues. This groove is called the *gingival sulcus* (see page 142). It surrounds each and every tooth. The depth of the gingival sulcus will vary; ideally it should not be more than 1 to 2 mm in depth. Within the gingival sulcus the tissue is not keratinized. At the bottom of the sulcus, and sealed to the tooth, is the epithelial attachment, which extends down toward the cemento-enamel junction. Attrition and/or disease often cause the epithelial attachment to migrate below the cemento-enamel junction and along the root of the tooth (see page 143).

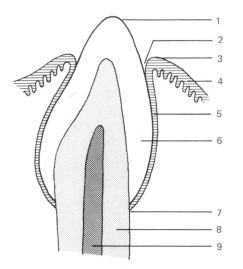

Diagrammatic illustration of the attached epithelial cuff and gingival sulcus at an early stage of tooth eruption. (1) Enamel on crown of erupting tooth; (2) gingival sulcus; (3) gingival margin; (4) oral epithelium; (5) attached gingiva; (6) enamel; (7) cemento-enamel junction; (8) dentin; (9) pulp.

Free Gingiva. Free gingiva is a fairly mobile tissue that surrounds but is not attached directly to the tooth. It extends from the bottom of the gingival sulcus upward to the gingival margin. It is separated from the tooth by the gingival sulcus whose outer surface is keratinized.

Gingival Margin. The gingival margin is the crest of the free gingiva, or the uppermost edge.

Free Gingival Groove. The free gingival groove is a shallow groove running parallel to the gingival margin and approximately 1 mm below it. It divides the free gingiva from the attached gingiva.

Attached Gingiva. The attached gingiva is the gingiva that is attached directly to the cementum and the alveolar process. It may be anywhere from 1 mm to 8 mm in width. It has no submucous layer. It extends from the free gingival groove to the mucogingival border (junction). It is stippled. In the attached gingiva, and between the teeth, there appear slight vertical depressions called *interdental grooves*. These vertical grooves are due to depressions between eminences in the alveolar process that covers the roots of the teeth.

Interdental Papillae. Interdental papillae form the gingival tissue that fills the triangular spaces between the teeth. Between the lingual and facial surface of each papilla is a concavity. This concavity is called a *col*.

Mucogingival Border. The mucogingival border is a scalloped border between the gingiva and the alveolar mucosa. The change in appearance from the gingiva to the mucosa is dramatic, as the color of the gingiva is pale pink and the mucosa is red and shiny. This dramatic dividing line occurs on the facial and lingual of the mandible, but it is not apparent on the palatal side of the maxillae.

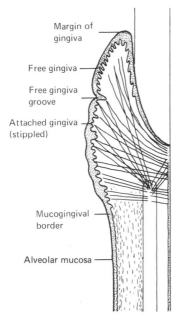

Margin of gingiva

Free gingiva

Free gingiva groove

Attached gingiva (stippled)

Mucogingival border

Alveolar mucosa

Diagram illustrating the difference between the free gingiva, the attached gingiva, and the alveolar mucosa.

Marginal Gingivitis. Marginal gingivitis is one of the most common forms of gingival inflammation. It is found in young children as well as in adults. This is a condition caused by poor oral hygiene, and when all irritations are removed, the condition will clear up quickly.

Calculus. Calculus is often the cause of marginal gingivitis. Supragingival (above the gingival margin) calculus formation varies from individual to individual. It is most frequently found on the lingual surface of the lower anterior teeth and opposite the openings of the salivary glands, particularly on the buccal surface of the posterior teeth. It is usually light yellow in color, unless stained by tobacco, tea, or coffee. Subgingival (below the gingival margin) calculus may be found anywhere and is usually darker in color and much harder than the supragingival type. It is important that the dental auxiliary recognize the supragingival calculus when performing an intra-oral examination. The subgingival calculus too should be detected, either with an explorer (dental instrument) or by radiographic examination.

The diagrammatic illustrations below show the location of the surface characteristics of the gingiva that are important to the dental auxiliary.

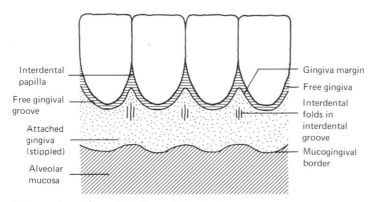

The surface characteristics of the gingiva.

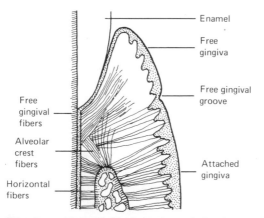

Drawing of longitudinal section of the free and attached gingiva separated by the free gingival groove. Note the free gingival, the alveolar crest, and the horizontal fibers.

NEW WORDS

Buccal: Toward the cheek.

Col: An indentation or depression on the crest of the interdental papilla where it meets the point of tooth contact.

SELF—TEST

1. Define the word *keratininzed*. _____

2. What color is gingiva when healthy? _____

3. Where is the gingival sulcus? _____

4. Approximately how deep will it be when in a healthy condition? _____

5. Give the general location of the epithelial attachment. _____

6. Give the location of the free gingiva. _____

7. Where is the gingival margin? _____

8. What is the free gingival groove? _____

9. What is the appearance of attached gingiva? Give the term for the vertical grooves between the teeth in the attached gingiva. _____

_____

10. What is the gingival tissue that fills the triangular spaces between the teeth called? What is the col? _____

_____

11. Describe the mucogingival border. _____

12. Is marginal gingivitis common? _____

13. Describe the difference between supragingival calculus and subgingival calculus. _____

_____

14. Where is the most calculus found in the mouth? Why? _____

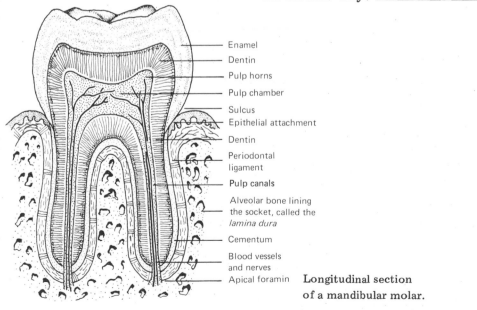

- Enamel
- Dentin
- Pulp horns
- Pulp chamber
- Sulcus
- Epithelial attachment
- Dentin
- Periodontal ligament
- Pulp canals
- Alveolar bone lining the socket, called the *lamina dura*
- Cementum
- Blood vessels and nerves
- Apical foramin

Longitudinal section of a mandibular molar.

145

4

Dental Anatomy

Nature has given all animals some means of tearing off and breaking down food into easily swallowed and digested bits. One of the devices that nature has provided for this necessary function of eating is teeth. The number of teeth, their size, and their form differ within the animal groups. Depending on individual need, some animals have no teeth; some, only one; and some have many. Man, the most advanced species of the animal kingdom, has a heterodont (het'-er-o-dont") dentition, that is, teeth of different shapes. During a lifetime, man has only two complete sets of teeth: (1) the 20 primary or deciduous teeth, and (2) the 32 permanent teeth; whereas other species may have a continuous supply. For example, when an alligator loses a tooth, another erupts to replace it. Man is not so fortunate; when teeth are lost, he must rely on artificial replacements, and these have seldom proved to be as satisfictory as the ones nature provided.

The dental auxiliary has a vital part in the dentist's plan to prevent loss of teeth, and must enthusiastically endorse, teach, and practice preventive dentistry. Recently, many states have changed their dental practice acts so as to allow dental auxiliaries to place restorative or temporary material in teeth damaged by dental caries. In order to perform these functions, it is vital for the student to learn tooth anatomy and to study, in detail, the crown of each tooth and, in particular, the occlusal anatomy of the posterior teeth.

The information presented in the following pages is much the same as material found in any study of dental anatomy. However, it is presented in a more simplified manner than that found in most such textbooks, in order to make it easy for a new student to grasp.

146

LANDMARKS

Anatomical and Clinical Crown

All fully developed teeth have a crown as well as a root portion. The crown portion is that part covered with enamel that extends from the cemento-enamel junction to the biting or crushing surfaces of the teeth. The root portion is covered with cementum and is embedded in the jaw; it extends from the cemento-enamel junction to the apex of the tooth. The cemento-enamel junction is sometimes referred to as the *cervical line.*

The crown portion is divided into two portions: (1) the portion that can be seen in the oral cavity, extending from the gingival margin to the biting or crushing surface of a tooth, is called the *clinical crown*; and (2) the portion that is covered by enamel (the entire crown) is called the *anatomical crown* (see following figure).

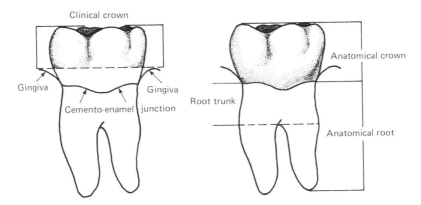

Buccal view of the mandibular left first molar.

Classifications

Teeth may be classified in five different ways:

1. The Arches
2. The Quadrants
3. Functions
4. Anterior group
   Centrals
   Laterals
   Canines
5. Posterior group
   Premolars
   Molars

Four of the above classifications—the arch, the quadrants, and the anterior and posterior groups—are shown on the illustration on page 148:

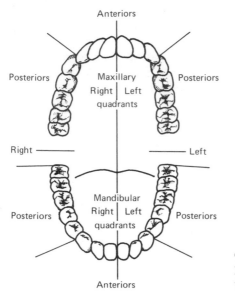

The maxillary and the mandibular arches in the permanent dentition.

The Arches. There are two arches in the mouth; the maxillary (upper) arch, and the mandibular (lower) arch.

The Quadrants. The maxillary and the mandibular arches are divided into two equal halves by the midline, which results in a total of four quadrants. In the adult dentition there are eight teeth in each quadrant, and in the deciduous dentition there are five teeth in each quadrant. However, during the time of transition from deciduous to adult dentition, the number of teeth at any given time, in the deciduous dentition, will vary according to the age of the child. One example would be the first permanent molar that erupts when a child is about the age of six. At this time there would be six teeth in that quadrant where the eruption takes place.

Functions. Teeth may be classified according to their function. The anatomy of each tooth within each classification is designed to perform a given function efficiently. In the normal adult or deciduous dentitions, the buccal cusps (pointed projections) of the maxillary posterior teeth extend over the buccal cusps of the mandibular posterior teeth, permitting the lingual cusps of the maxillary posterior teeth to fit into the central fossae of the mandibular teeth. This arrangement assists in stabilizing the arches and also creates surfaces that perform as a mortar and pestle in the grinding and pulverizing of food. Generally, the anterior teeth do not have contact and serve only to incise food.

  Incisors. The incisors, both centrals and laterals, have sharp cutting edges (incisal edges) to permit the biting or cutting of food. This is why they are called *incisors,* for *to incise* means "to cut."

Canines. The canine teeth, at the corners of each quadrant, are the longest and strongest teeth in the mouth. They have one labial cusp that serves to grasp, tear, or hold food. They too, like the central and lateral incisors, may be used to bite or cut food. The strength of the canines and the length of their roots serve to help support the central and lateral incisors during functional stress.

Premolars. The premolars are sometimes called *bicuspids*, but this term, meaning "two cusps," is not entirely accurate because there may be one or three cusps present. Therefore, the term *premolar*, meaning that these teeth are situated in front of the molars, is more correct. The premolars in each quadrant are designed to assist the canine teeth to grasp and hold, and to assist the molars to grind, crush, or pulverize food.

Molars. There are three molars in each quadrant of the adult dentition. Each molar has broad surfaces with several points of contact, making an efficient tool for crushing food to bits.

Anterior, Middle, and Posterior Segments. Most texts divide the teeth into anterior and posterior segments, as noted in the preceding figure and outline; but tooth alignment should really be divided into three segments: anterior, middle, and posterior. The anterior segment includes the central and lateral incisors, ending at the labial ridge (center of the labial cusp) of the canine. The middle segment includes the distal surface of the canine, the premolars, and the buccal ridge of the mesiobuccal cusps of the first molars. The posterior extends from the mesiobuccal cusps of the first molar to the distal surface of the third molar. This arrangement gives credence to the belief that the canines and the first molar serve as supports for both arches.[1]

Arrangement of Teeth

The teeth, both deciduous and permanent, are arranged in the oral cavity to provide maximum efficiency during the taking in and the preparation of food for deglutition, digestion, and absorption. The teeth in both the maxillary and the mandibular arches articulate in such a manner that they not only assist in the preparation of food for digestion; but also each tooth, in turn, assists in supporting its neighbor. The loss of even one tooth will disrupt the efficiency of these functions.

All permanent molars are nonsuccedaneous teeth because there are no primary teeth preceding them into the oral cavity. All anterior teeth and the permanent premolars are succedaneous because there are 10 primary teeth in each arch that precede them.

There are 20 succedaneous teeth in all. The names of all teeth correspond to those shown in the left maxillary quadrant on page 150.

[1] Russell C. Wheeler, *Dental Anatomy Physiology and Occlusion*, 4th ed. (Philadelphia: W. B. Saunders Company, 1974), p. 419.

The diagrammatic illustration below names the teeth and identifies those teeth that are succedaneous.

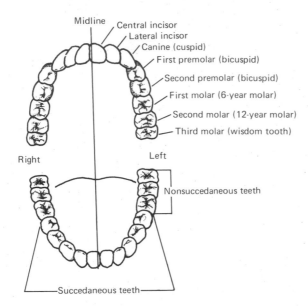

Location and names of teeth in the permanent dentition.

Tooth Surfaces

Each tooth in the oral cavity has five surfaces. Any tooth surface facing toward the midline is called *mesial*. And any tooth surface facing away from the midline is called *distal*. The biting surface on the anterior teeth is referred to as *incisal*. The chewing surface on the posterior teeth is referred to as *occlusal*. When referring to the surface of the anterior teeth that face the lips, one uses the term *labial*. When referring to the surface of the posterior teeth facing the cheeks, one uses the word *buccal*.

In reference to all tooth surfaces facing the vestibule, the term used is *facial*. In reference to all tooth surfaces facing the tongue, the term used is *lingual*. The *vestibule* is the space between the cheek and the teeth and between the lips and the teeth in both the maxillae and the mandible (see figure on page 151).

Thus each tooth has five surfaces as listed below.

Anterior teeth surfaces	*Posterior teeth surfaces*
Mesial	Mesial
Distal	Distal
Lingual	Lingual
Labial	Buccal
Incisal	Occlusal

These five surfaces are depicted in the following two diagrams.

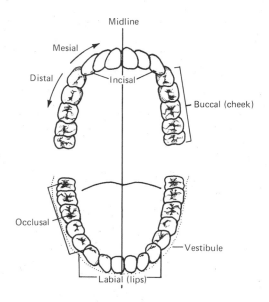

The location of each tooth surface.

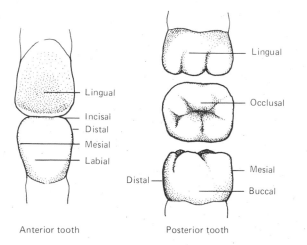

Anterior tooth   Posterior tooth

Tooth surfaces.

Division of the Tooth Surfaces into Thirds

To identify and locate an exact area of the crown or root of a tooth, each may be divided by imaginary lines into thirds. The crown may be divided in several ways, but the root is only divided into cervical, middle, and apical thirds (see figure on page 152).

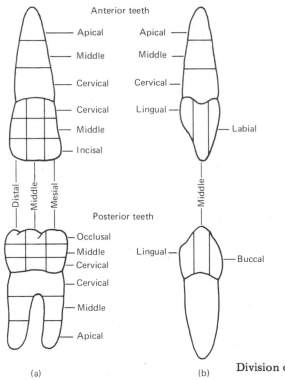

Anterior teeth

— Apical   Apical —

— Middle   Middle —

— Cervical   Cervical —

— Cervical   Lingual —

— Middle   — Labial

— Incisal

Distal — Middle — Mesial   Middle

Posterior teeth

— Occlusal   Lingual —

— Middle   — Buccal

— Cervical

— Cervical

— Middle

— Apical

(a)   (b)   Division of the tooth into thirds.

Line and Point Angles

In order to identify certain areas with accuracy, names are given to the line and point angles on the crowns of the teeth. These angles are junctions on the crowns where different surfaces meet. A *line angle* represents the junction of *two surfaces*, such as the mesial and labial surfaces of an anterior tooth. This junction is called the *mesiolabial line angle*. A *point angle* represents the meeting point of *three surfaces*, such as the mesial, labial, and incisal surfaces. This angle is called the *mesiolabioincisal point angle*. You will note that whenever you are combining the names of surfaces, an "o" is substituted for the "al," making the name change from *mesial* to *mesio*, etc.

The line and point angles are used as points of reference to identify and locate exact areas that the dentist and auxiliary will refer to when charting and planning the restoration of teeth in the oral cavity (see illustration on page 153).

Contact Areas and Embrasures

The contact area is the area on the mesial and distal surfaces of a tooth that contacts the adjacent tooth. There is contact, mesially and distally, on all teeth except the third molar, which has only mesial contact with the second molar. If no contact is made with the adjacent tooth, the space created

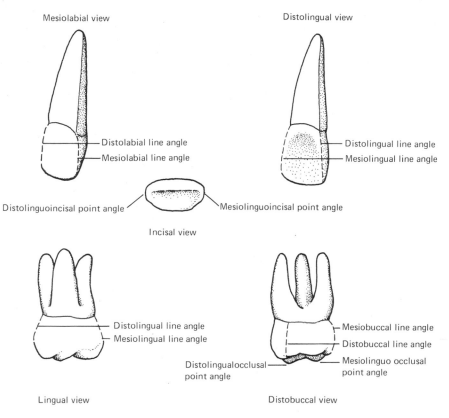

Mesiolabial view

Distolingual view

Distolabial line angle
Mesiolabial line angle

Distolingual line angle
Mesiolingual line angle

Distolinguoincisal point angle

Mesiolinguoincisal point angle

Incisal view

Distolingual line angle
Mesiolingual line angle

Mesiobuccal line angle
Distobuccal line angle

Distolingualocclusal point angle

Mesiolinguo occlusal point angle

Lingual view

Distobuccal view

Line and point angles.

is referred to as a *diastema* (dī'-a-stē'-ma). In order to locate contact areas, the teeth should be observed from the facial, incisal, and occlusal aspects. These areas, when observed from the facial aspect, will be found in the occlusal or incisal third of most teeth. However, some of the teeth have mesial or distal contact in the middle third or a combination of middle and occlusal third. In the anterior teeth from the incisal aspect the contact areas appear almost as points, while in the posterior teeth they are broader and flatter. See figure below.

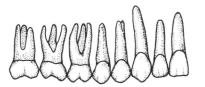

From the facial and lingual aspects, embrasures can be seen just below the contact area. They appear as triangular spaces and are usually filled with gingival tissue. From the occlusal and incisal aspect, triangular spaces can be seen; their flaring form serves to make the teeth somewhat self-cleansing.

These embrasures and contact areas protect the gingival tissues from trauma during the mastication of food. See figure below.

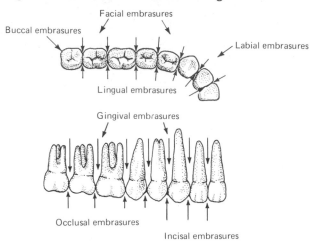

Tooth Numbering

To identify the location and to chart conditions of individual teeth, it was found necessary to give each tooth a number. Over the years many methods of tooth numbering evolved, and some are still in use today. However, in 1968 the Council on Dental Education announced that the American Dental Association's House of Delegates had developed a standardized system of tooth numbering called the "Universal Method" and suggested that this system be taught in all dental auxiliary curriculums.

It is important that dental auxiliaries have a thorough knowledge of tooth numbering, because charting and recording of the patient's dental conditions are the only record a dentist has for reference after the intial examination. From these records he must plan his procedures for completing the case.

Most dental charts divide the mouth vertically into the right and left sides by the midline (midsaggital plane). It is again divided horizontally into upper and lower, or maxillary and mandibular arches, by the occlusal plane. See figure below.

Two methods of tooth identification are shown in the diagrammatic illustration below.

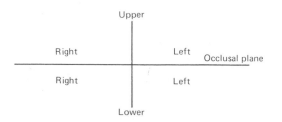

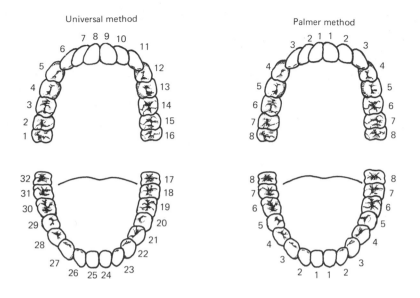

Universal method

Palmer method

Tooth numbering of the permanent dentition.

SELF—TEST

1. The term *heterodont* means: one tooth, multiple sets, different shapes. (Circle one.)

2. The complete primary dentition has how many teeth? _____

3. The complete permanent dentition has how many teeth? _____

4. Give another term for cemento-enamel junction. _____

5. How many anterior teeth are there in the maxillary arch? In the mandibular arch? _____

6. How many posterior teeth are there in the mandibular arch? In the maxillary arch? _____

7. What do we mean by *mixed dentition*? _____

8. The normal permanent dentition will contain how many succedaneous teeth? _____

9. What is the chief function of the incisors? _____

10. What is the chief function of the molars? _____

11. What is the chief function of the canines? _____

12. The valley that encircles each arch between the teeth and the cheeks and the lips is called the _____ .

13. When referring to *all* surfaces facing the cheeks and lips, what term is used? _____

14. When referring to all surfaces facing the tongue, what term is used? _____

15. To identify and locate exact areas of the crown or root of a tooth, the teeth may be divided by imaginary lines into: quadrants, sixths, thirds, halves. (Circle one.)

16. The junction of three surfaces of a tooth is called a _____ .

17. The junction of two surfaces of a tooth is called a _____ .

18. Locate the contact areas on the drawing below.

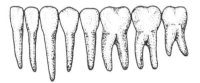

19. Locate the anatomical crown, clinical crown, cementoenamel junction, anatomical root, and the root trunk on the figures below.

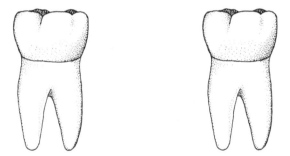

20. Locate the five surfaces on each of the teeth below.

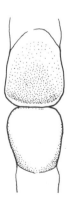
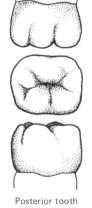

Anterior tooth   Posterior tooth

21. Define *diastema*. _____

22. Locate and name the embrasures on the drawings below.

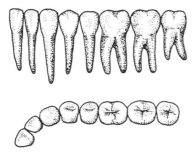

23. Number the teeth, according to the Universal Method, on the drawing below.

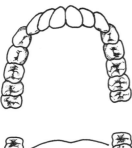

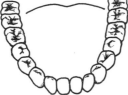

TERMS USED IN DENTISTRY

Angle. A figure formed by the coming together of two parts. A right angle is 90°, and anything less is an acute angle, and anything more is an obtuse angle.

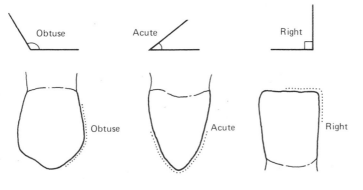

Angles.

Axial. Meaning "long," and in dentistry pertaining to the long axis of the tooth.

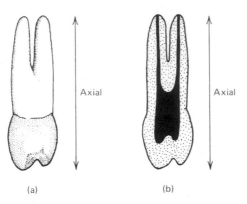

(a)   (b)

Maxillary first premolar. (a) Mesial view; (b) buccolingual cross section.

Cingulum. The cingulum is a smooth convexity just below the cervical line on the lingual surface. It is found only on the cervical third of all anterior teeth.

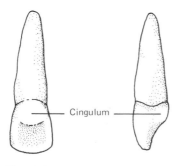

Cingulum

Lingual view   Mesial view   **Central incisor.**

Concave. A hollow or a void.

Concave

Convex. A curved or rounded form.

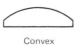

Convex

Cusp. A cusp is an elevation or mound on the biting surface of the crown of a tooth.

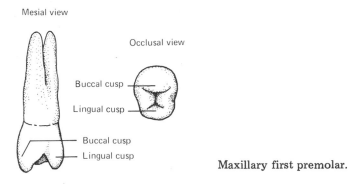

Mesial view

Occlusal view

Buccal cusp

Lingual cusp

Buccal cusp

Lingual cusp

Maxillary first premolar.

Fossa. A fossa is an irregular depression or concavity. Such depressions may be found on the lingual surface of the anterior teeth and on the occlusal surface of the posterior teeth.

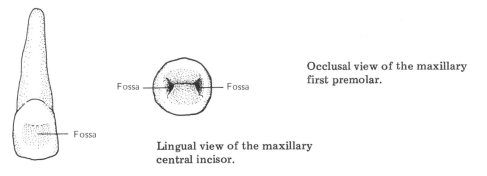

Fossa — — Fossa

Occlusal view of the maxillary first premolar.

— Fossa

Lingual view of the maxillary central incisor.

Furcation. Furcation means "forked"; "branching like a fork." Furcations will be found on all multirooted teeth. *Trifurcation* means divided into three branches as in teeth having three roots. *Bifurcation* means divided into two branches as in teeth having two roots. See diagrams below.

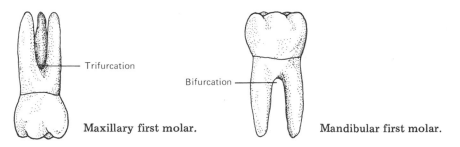

— Trifurcation

Bifurcation —

Maxillary first molar.   Mandibular first molar.

Grooves. A groove is either a furrow, a channel, or a rut. In dentistry there are developmental grooves and supplemental grooves. See figure on page 158.

Developmental Grooves. Developmental grooves occur between parts of the crown or root; they are shallow grooves that mark the junction between primary parts.

Supplemental Grooves. Supplemental grooves are very shallow grooves on the occlusal surface of posterior teeth.

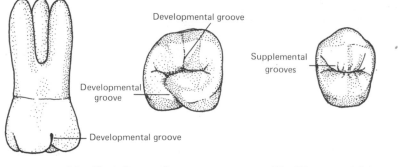

Maxillary first molar.   Maxillary second premolar.

Lobes. A lobe represents a developing cusp. It is the primary center of formation. The lobes eventually coalesce (grow together) and form the crowns of the teeth. There are generally four lobes on the anterior teeth (centrals, laterals and canines), the premolars, the second molars, and the third molars. There are five lobes on the maxillary first molar, the mandibular first molar, and the mandibular second premolar. Numbers of lobes are indicated on figures below.

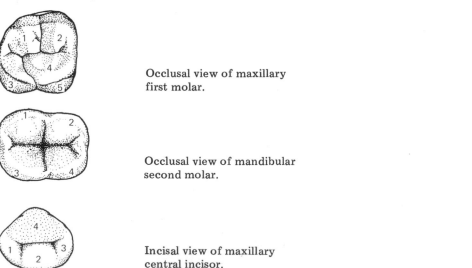

Occlusal view of maxillary first molar.

Occlusal view of mandibular second molar.

Incisal view of maxillary central incisor.

Mamelons. Mamelons are small rounded prominences on the incisal edge of the maxillary and mandibular lateral incisors and central incisors. They mark the termination of each of the three labial lobes. On newly erupted teeth the mamelons are quite prominent. Generally, they are worn away, quite soon, through the incising of food.

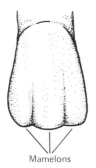

Mamelons Labial view of maxillary central incisor.

Pit. A pit is a very small depression located at the junction of developmental grooves or at the end of a developmental groove.

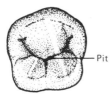

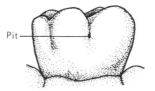

Occlusal view of mandibular second premolar.

Buccal view of mandibular first molar.

Proximal Surface. The proximal surface is the surface next to an adjacent tooth. All teeth with the exception of the third molar, have proximal surfaces.

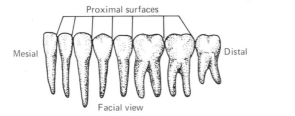

Facial view.

Ridge. A ridge is a long or linear elevation on the surface of a tooth. It is named for its location.

Buccal Ridge. The buccal ridge is a ridge extending down the center of the buccal surface of the premolars from the cervical line to the occlusal surface.

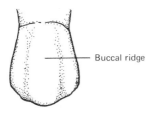

Buccal view of the maxillary second premolar.

Cusp Ridge. The cusp ridge marks the height of each cusp on the posterior teeth. The cusps divide the buccal surface from the occlusal surface.

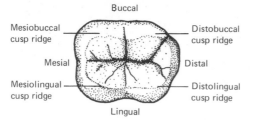

Occlusal view of mandibular first molar.

Labial Ridge. The labial ridge extends down the center of the labial surface of the canines. See figure below.

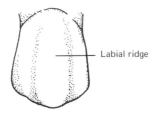

Labial view of the maxillary canine.

Marginal Ridges. Marginal ridges are the rounded elevations of enamel found on the mesial and distal surfaces of all teeth. On the anterior teeth, the ridges are located on the lingual surface; on the posterior teeth, the ridges are located on the occlusal surface.

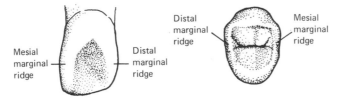

Lingual view of the maxillary lateral incisor.

Occlusal view of the maxillary first premolar.

Oblique Ridge. The oblique ridge is found on the maxillary molars, being generally more pronounced on the first maxillary molar than on the second maxillary molar. It is a slanting ridge; hence the term *oblique.*

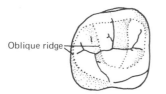

Occlusal view of the maxillary first molar.

Triangular Ridges. Triangular ridges descend from the tips of the cusps to the central groove on the occlusal surface of the posterior teeth. These ridges are named after the cusps where they are located (see diagrams below).

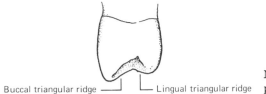

Buccal triangular ridge ——   —— Lingual triangular ridge   Mesial view of the maxillary first premolar.

Transverse Ridge. A transverse ridge is formed when two triangular ridges join as they cross the occlusal surface of a posterior tooth. See figure below.

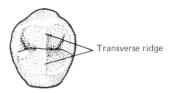

Transverse ridge

Occlusal view of the maxillary first premolar.

Tubercle. The cusp of Carabelli, or fifth cusp, on the maxillary first molar is sometimes referred to as a *tubercle.* A tubercle is a small knoblike prominence. At times the cusp on the lingual surface of the mandibular first premolar is so small that it, too, is referred to as a tubercle.

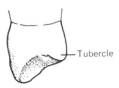
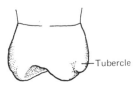

Tubercle   Tubercle

Mesial view of a maxillary first molar.

Mesial view of mandibular first premolar.

Sulcus. A sulcus is a long depression between ridges and cusps (see figure below). It inclines to meet at an angle, where it joins with a developmental groove.

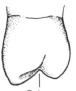

Sulcus   Mesial view of the maxillary first premolar.

1. Identify the geometric forms below.

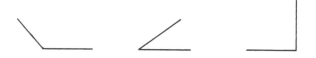

2. Indicate the long axis of the tooth on the illustration below.

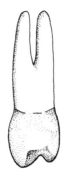

3. Indicate the location of the cingulum on the illustration below.

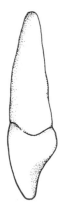

4. Define *concave* and *convex*. _____

5. Define *cusps* and tell where they are located. _____

_____

6. Define *fossae*. Are they found on all teeth? _____

7. Define *furcation* and tell where it may be found in the dentition. _____

_____

8. On the illustration below, indicate by letter the following: (a) developmental groove; (b) supplemental groove; (c) the fifth lobe.

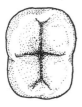

Occlusal view of the maxillary first molar.

9. Which teeth have four lobes, and which have five? _____

10. Define *mamelons* and tell where they are located. _____

11. Define *pits* and tell where they are generally found. _____

12. Define *proximal.* _____

13. On the illustrations below, indicate by letter the following ridges: (a) buccal ridge; (b) mesiobuccal cusp ridge; (c) distobuccal cusp ridge; (d) marginal ridge; (e) oblique ridge; (f) transverse ridge; (g) triangular ridge.

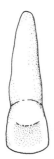

Maxillary canine.

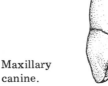

Maxillary first premolar.

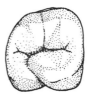

Maxillary first molar.

14. Define *tubercle.* _____

15. Indicate the sulcus on the drawing below.

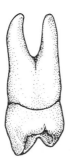

Maxillary first premolar.

Lying within the upper and lower jaw, at the time of birth, are 44 teeth in various stages of development. Twenty of these teeth are the child's first, or primary, teeth; and the balance are permanent teeth that will begin to erupt when the child reaches the age of six or seven. The primary mandibular central incisors are usually the first to erupt when the child is between six and seven months; however, as with all things in nature, anomalies do occur, and occasionally a child will be born with one or more teeth already present in the oral cavity. These premature teeth, due to their incomplete root development, are not retained for long. Also occasionally the first deciduous teeth will not appear until a child is in the eleventh or twelfth month, causing the parents great anxiety. This, however, should not be viewed as a cause for alarm.

The first 20 teeth are frequently not considered to be of great importance by parents, and they are thought of, and referred to, as just baby teeth or temporary teeth. This is a great tragedy because the primary teeth are very important to a child's health; they are needed during the growing years from five to twelve for normal jaw development, speech, mastication of food, esthetics, and space maintenance to permit the succeeding permanent teeth to erupt normally.

During the child's sixth year, the first permanent molars begin to erupt. Therefore this is the beginning of a period of mixed dentition, as there are both permanent and primary teeth present in the oral cavity. This stage will continue until the child is about twelve. In general, the primary and the permanent teeth appear to be similar; however, it is not too difficult to distinguish between them. The deciduous (or primary) teeth are usually much whiter and smaller with shorter crowns, than the permanent teeth. Also, in the primary teeth, the pulp chambers are larger, and the roots are rather long, slender, and widespread; and there is little or no root trunk, in comparison to the permanent teeth.

The roots of the primary teeth develop and become completely formed after the tooth has erupted into the oral cavity; this takes about one year. After one to two years more, the roots of the primary teeth will begin to resorb to permit exfoliation (casting off) of the crown. This will allow space for the erupting permanent teeth. During resorption of the root there will be periods of inactivity to allow reattachment of the periodontal fibers. Also during this time the primary tooth will have alternate periods of tightening and loosening until the crown has been shed and the permanent tooth enters the oral cavity.

After the child is two years of age, the primary teeth should be in normal alignment and in occlusion. As the jaws continue to grow, a diastema (space) will develop between some of the teeth, usually with the greater separation occurring between the anteriors. This is a normal condition.

All teeth erupt into the oral cavity at various times—ranging from five

months to 25 years or even later. Below is an approximate time chart of the
eruption times of the deciduous teeth.

Primary Teeth	*Age at Eruption*
4 central incisors	6th to 9th month
4 lateral incisors	7th to 10th month
4 first molars	12th to 14th month
4 canines	16th to 20th month
4 second molars	20th to 25th month

The following illustrations of the labial and occlusal aspects of the
deciduous dentition names and locates the primary teeth. Also shown is one
method of numbering primary teeth so they may be readily identified. The
names of all teeth correspond to those shown in the maxillary left quadrant
in the figure above.

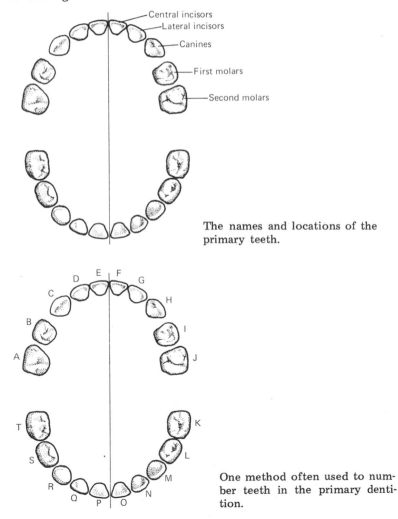

The names and locations of the primary teeth.

One method often used to number teeth in the primary dentition.

SELF—TEST

1. When do a child's permanent teeth begin to erupt? _____

2. Which teeth are the first to erupt in the primary dentition? _____

3. How important is it to care for the teeth in the primary dentition? Why?
_____

4. When do the first permanent molars erupt? Will there be both permanent and primary teeth present in the oral cavity at that time? _____

5. What term is used when both primary and permanent teeth are present?
_____

6. Name two things that would help one to distinguish between the primary and the permanent teeth. _____

7. How long does it take after eruption for the roots of the primary teeth to become fully formed? _____

8. What happens to the root eventually that will permit the tooth to be exfoliated? _____

9. Define *diastema*. _____

10. What age is the child when the primary second molars erupt? _____

11. How are primary teeth numbered or lettered to permit identification when charting an oral exam? _____

PERMANENT DENTITION

The first permanent teeth to erupt into the oral cavity are the six-year molars. They are given this name because they generally erupt during the child's sixth year. They erupt posterior to the deciduous molars and are frequently mistaken by parents to be deciduous teeth. The permanent mandibular and the permanent maxillary central incisors often erupt about the same time. The eruption of all permanent teeth continues as the deciduous teeth are exfoliated and as the jaws develop enough to provide more space. This results in a very mixed dentition. This pattern of eruption continues until a child is about 14, and the entire succedaneous dentition is in place. The

Eruptions Times for Permanent Teeth

Central incisor	6 to 7 years	
Lateral incisor	7 to 8 years	
Canine	9 to 10 years	Succedaneous teeth
Mandibular first premolar	10 to 12 years	
Mandibular second premolar	11 to 12 years	
Mandibular first molar	6 to 7 years	
Mandibular second molar	11 to 13 years	Nonsuccedaneous teeth
Mandibular third molar	17 to 21 years	

168

approximate eruption times of all permanent teeth should be studied, as often it is the auxiliary that must answer a patient's questions concerning this process.

It should be remembered that the mandibular teeth usually precede the maxillary teeth into the oral cavity, and that the roots of all teeth are completed approximately two or more years after eruption takes place.

The anatomy of the crown of each tooth in the right quadrant of the maxillary and mandibular arches and the distinguishing features of each will be covered. The roots of the teeth will be only briefly discussed, since an in-depth study is not considered necessary to meet the objectives of this chapter.

The basic function of the root of a tooth is to support the crown. The roots of the teeth are suspended in the alveoli. They are covered with cementum and are held in place by the attachment of periodontal ligaments to the cementum on one side and to the alveolar bone of the alveoli on the other. The permanent teeth may have one, two, three, or more roots. Normally those having *one root* are the centrals, laterals, canines, maxillary second premolars, and the mandibular first and second premolars. Those teeth normally having *two roots* are the maxillary first premolars and the mandibular first and second molars. The teeth that normally have *three roots* are the maxillary first and second molars. Third molars, both maxillary and mandibular, are apt to have anywhere from one to seven or eight roots, or their roots may be fused together to resemble one.

Although the permanent teeth have only one, two, or three roots, accessory canals may be found in some of the roots. For instance, the mesial root of the mandibular molars has a mesiolingual canal as well as a mesiobuccal canal.

In order to prepare oneself to restore damaged tooth structure to its original form, the crowns of all teeth should be carefully studied and then carved in wax, soap, or plaster. If possible, you should obtain models of teeth made from ivoryine (synthetic material) or extracted teeth in which cavities have been prepared. Wax can then be melted into the preparation and carved, restoring the tooth's original anatomy. This wax can then be removed from the preparation and the entire procedure done over and over until perfection is obtained.

Accuracy, when restoring the occlusal surface of a tooth, cannot be stressed too much. Correct relationship of mandibular teeth to maxillary teeth must be preserved or *malocclusion* (bad occlusion) will result, causing unnecessary discomfort or possible pain for the patient.

When carving the occlusal surfaces, remember that the grooves establish proper anatomy. Keep them definite but smooth, so that they may be easily cleaned. Be certain to restore marginal ridges correctly in order to convey food in the proper direction, or impaction of food will result in that area.

Many things contribute to a healthy mouth and proper occlusal contact, including correct intercuspal relationships and good mesial and distal contacts. Careful restoration of carious teeth will help maintain the functional relationship of teeth and will contribute extensively to a patient's good oral health.

SELF—TEST

1. Which of the permanent teeth are the first teeth to erupt into the oral cavity? When? _____

2. Are there other permanent teeth that might erupt at the same time? Explain. _____

3. What is the term given to the period when there are both permanent and deciduous teeth present? _____

4. How many roots do each of the following have?

Maxillary Teeth		*Mandibular Teeth*	
Centrals	_____	Centrals	_____
Laterals	_____	Laterals	_____
Canines	_____	Canines	_____
First premolars	_____	First premolars	_____
Second premolars	_____	Second premolars	_____
First molars	_____	First molars	_____
Second molars	_____	Second molars	_____

5. Do some of the roots have more than one pulp canal? Give one example.
_____

6. Name three things that will contribute to a healthy mouth and proper occlusal contact. _____
_____

7. Do the maxillary teeth erupt before the mandibular teeth? _____

ANATOMY OF THE INDIVIDUAL TEETH IN THE MAXILLARY AND MANDIBULAR RIGHT QUADRANTS

The illustrations on the following pages show the geometric form and describe the anatomy of the crown of each tooth in the maxillary and mandibular right quadrants. These illustrations and descriptions will be helpful when reproducing the form and anatomical characteristics of teeth being restored in cement or amalgam.

The illustration shows the occlusal anatomy on the biting and chewing surfaces of all teeth in both arches.

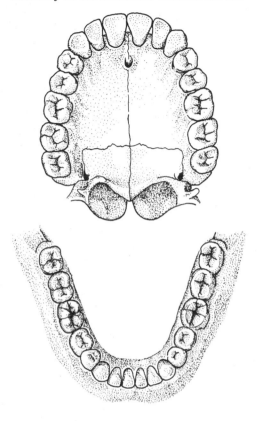

Occlusal view of the upper and lower permanent teeth.

Geometric Outline Forms

When studying the crowns of teeth, one should be aware of the geometric outline forms present. Most crowns fit into one of these three shapes.

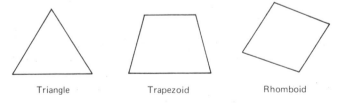

Triangle   Trapezoid   Rhomboid

Triangle: A figure with three sides and three angles.
Trapezoid: A plane four-sided figure with only two sides parallel.
Rhomboid: A parallelogram in which the angles are oblique and the adjacent sides are unequal.

The size of the tooth, its location in the maxillae or mandible, whether anterior or posterior, and whether the crown is observed from the mesial, distal, facial, or lingual aspect will determine the size and the shape of the geometric form. The following three figures illustrate the triangle, trapezoid, and rhomboid shapes of crowns, respectively.

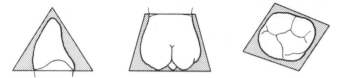

Variations in human dentition may occur, as a result of: (1) the number of lobes developing, (2) the shapes of the developed lobes, (3) the arrangement of the lobes, and (4) the arrangement of the lobes in relation to each other.

Nature has designed our teeth to allow self-cleansing action, strength, and stability; to establish correct occlusion for the proper mastication of food; and to maintain the oral tissues in good health.

Maxillary Central Incisors: Key Points to Observe

1. The crowns of the maxillary central incisors are shaped like a wedge or triangle when observed from the medial or distal aspect; but when viewed from the labial or lingual aspect, the crown shape is trapezoidal.
2. When viewed from the buccal aspect, the mesial surface appears nearly straight and slightly longer than the distal surface, which is more convex.
3. The incisal edge is usually straight in a mesiodistal direction, with but a slight curve toward the distal at the distoincisal angle. At times the middle third may be slightly longer than the mesial and distal thirds. There will be mamelons on newly erupted teeth. These are worn away through mastication as one grows older.
4. On the labial and lingual surface, the height of cervical curvature is toward the apex of the root, and the cervical line appears like a half moon.
5. There are two slight depressions (developmental grooves) on the labial surface. These depressions mark the joining of the three labial lobes.
6. The lingual surface of the crown is narrower than the labial surface.
7. The mesial and distal marginal ridges on the lingual surface are well-rounded.
8. The cingulum or lingual (4th) lobe is found on the lingual surface at the cervical line in the cervical third. This convexity extends down to the lingual fossa.
9. Four lobes make up the crown of this tooth.
10. The lingual fossa is fairly deep and lies between the marginal ridges, the cingulum, and the incisal edge. Sometimes a deep lingual pit is found at the junction of the cingulum and the fossa.
11. On the mesial and distal surfaces, the cervical line curves toward the incisal edge. It curves approximately 3.5 mm on the mesial surface and 2.5 mm on the distal surface.

12. There is one root that is usually inclined toward the distal. It is straight and conical.

Illustrated below are five views of the maxillary right central incisor. Study these illustrations and the key points on the preceding page; then take the self-test that follows.

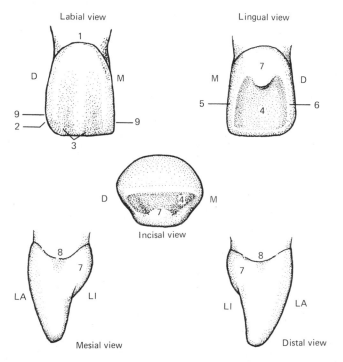

Views of the right maxillary central incisor. D, distal; M, mesial; LA, labial; LI, lingual. (1) Height of cervical curvature; (2) curvature of distoincisal angle; (3) labial developmental grooves (marking the joining of the lobes); (4) lingual fossa; (5) mesial marginal ridge; (6) distal marginal ridge; (7) cingulum; (8) cervical curvature (less on distal surface than on mesial surface); (9) contact areas—mesial surface close to the incisal and distal surfaces where the incisal and the middle thirds meet. *Note:* Contact areas are also called *crests of curvatures.*

SELF—TEST

1. What geometric forms may be applied to the maxillary central incisors, both on the labial and mesial surfaces? _____

_____

2. Is the mesioincisal angle or the distoincisal angle more curved? _____

3. When mamelons are present, what surface are they on? _____

4. Are mamelons present in the teeth of older persons? Give the reason for your answer. _____

_____

5. When looking at this tooth from the labial aspect, which is longest—the mesial surface or the distal surface? _____

6. How many lobes form the central incisor crown? _____

7. Occasionally one of the labial lobes may be longer than the others. To which lobe is this referring? _____

8. What embryological action caused the developmental grooves on the labial surface? _____

9. Where is the cingulum located on the central incisor? Be specific. _____
_____

10. Do the central incisors have marginal ridges? If so, on which surface or surfaces are they located? _____

11. What is meant by "height of curvature"? Be brief. _____
_____

12. Is the crown narrower on the lingual surface than on the labial surface?
_____

13. Where is the fossa on these teeth? _____

14. Does the height of curvature on the labial and lingual surfaces of the crown go toward the root or toward the incisal surface? _____

15. Does the depth of curvature on the mesial and distal surfaces go toward the apex of the root or toward the incisal surface? _____

16. Which has the greater depth of cervical curvature—the mesial surface or the distal surface? _____

17. Where is a fairly deep lingual pit sometimes found on the central incisor?
_____

18. The maxillary centrals have how many roots? Is there a distal curvature to the root? _____

Mandibular Central Incisors: Key Points to Observe

1. The crown of the mandibular central incisor is shaped like a triangle; when observed from the mesial or distal aspect, or from the labial or lingual aspect, it is shaped like a trapezoid.
2. The crown is generally smaller and narrower than the crown of any other tooth in the mouth. When observed from the labial or lingual aspect, it appears about one-half the width of the maxillary central incisor. However, when observed from the mesial or distal aspect, there is not much difference is shape, only in bulk.
3. The mesioincisal and distoincisal angles of this tooth form sharp right angles that taper down smoothly to the cervical line, being slightly convex at the incisal third. This is the contact area.
4. There are very few developmental grooves or lines on the labial surface,

and the lingual surface is almost smooth, with slight marginal ridges bordering a shallow fossa.

5. When the crown is observed from the mesial or distal aspect, a slight convexity is seen on the lingual surface at the cervical third. This is the cingulum.

6. The cervical curvature on the labial surface rounds gently toward the apex of the root.

7. The depth of cervical curvature on the mesial surface is about 1 mm, with the depth of curvature on the distal surface being slightly less.

8. The mandibular central incisors are the first teeth to erupt, and when newly erupted, they display three mamelons on the incisal edge, marking the labial lobes.

9. From the labial or lingual aspect, the root appears conical. When viewed from the mesial or distal aspect, it is somewhat wider and flatter, with a shallow depression extending most of the way from the cervical line to the apex.

Illustrated below are five views of the mandibular right central incisor. Study these illustrations and the key points on the preceding page; then take the self-test that follows.

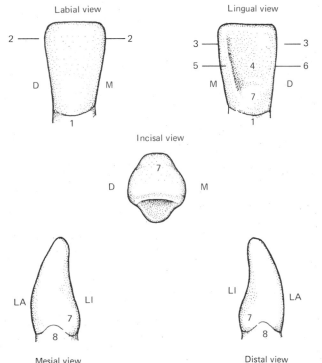

Views of the mandibular right central incisor. D, distal; M, mesial; LA, labial; LI, lingual. (1) Height of cervical curvature; (2) mesioincisal and distoincisal angles; (3) contact areas; (4) lingual fossa; (5) mesial marginal ridge; (6) distal marginal ridge; (7) cingulum; (8) cervical curvature.

1. Is the mandibular central incisor the smallest tooth in the mouth? _____

2. How many mandibular centrals are there? _____

3. Do these teeth erupt before any others? _____

4. Are the mesioincisal and the distoincisal angles very symmetrical? _____

5. In what third of the crown are the contact areas? _____

6. Is the lingual surface of the crowns of these teeth smooth and only slightly convex? Is the cingulum small? _____

7. Are the marginal ridges prominent or barely discernible? _____

8. What geometric shape does the crown of the mandibular central incisor resemble when viewed from the labial aspect? From the mesial aspect?

   _____

9. Does the labial surface appear almost flat when viewed from the mesial aspect? _____

10. Do these teeth display mamelons when newly erupted? _____

Maxillary Lateral Incisors: Key Points to Observe

1. The maxillary lateral incisors are much like the central incisors except in size. The crown appears shorter and narrower than that of the central incisor.
2. The distoincisal angle is well-rounded with a slight convexity that continues to the cervical line. The mesioincisal angle is also rounded but not as much as the distoincisal angle.
3. The crown is concave at the cervical line on the mesial surface; it then becomes convex to the incisal edge.
4. These teeth are the most varied in shape in the dentition. One or more may be missing or very abnormal in form, varying with the individual. Some anomalies are considered hereditary.
5. These teeth have a prominant cingulum at the cervical third of the lingual surface.
6. The mesial and distal marginal ridges on the lingual surface are very prominent. They are sturdy and well-rounded. The depth of the lingual fossa also produces a well-rounded incisal ridge.
7. Often there is a deep developmental groove on the cingulum. This most frequently is inclined toward the distal surface.
8. The depth of curvature at the cervical line is about 3 mm on the mesial surface, and on the distal surface it is about 2 mm.
9. Each tooth has one root that is straight and conical when viewed from the labial or the lingual aspect; however, when viewed from the mesial or the distal aspect, the root is somewhat flattened. It generally curves toward the distal side and terminates with a pointed apex.

Illustrated below are five views of the maxillary right lateral incisor. Study these illustrations and the key points on the preceding page; then take the self-test that follows.

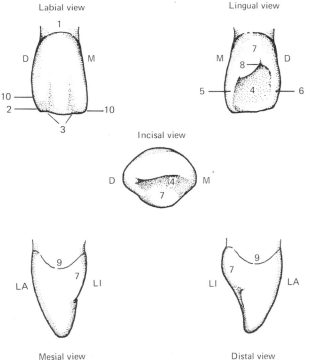

Views of the maxillary right lateral incisor. D, distal; M, mesial; LA, labial; LI, lingual. (1) Height of cervical curvature; (2) curvature of distoincisal angle; (3) labial developmental grooves; (4) lingual fossa; (5) mesial marginal ridge; (6) distal marginal ridge; (7) cingulum; (8) developmental groove; (9) cervical curvature; (10) contact areas.

SELF—TEST

1. In general form do the maxillary lateral incisors resemble the maxillary central incisors? _____

2. Is this tooth larger or smaller than the maxillary central incisor? _____

3. Is this tooth often deformed or missing? _____

4. Are the mesial and distal marginal ridges very prominent? If so, what would be the cause? _____

5. On which surface, and on what part of the crown, is the deep developmental groove (fissure) located? _____

6. Is the depth of cervical curvature on the mesial and distal surfaces of the crown more or less than on the maxillary central incisor? _____

7. How many roots does this tooth have? _____

Mandibular Lateral Incisors: Key Points to Observe

1. The mandibular lateral incisors closely resemble the mandibular central incisors. When observed from the labial or the lingual aspect, the crown is trapezoidal in shape; and when viewed from the mesial or distal aspect, the crown is triangular in shape.
2. These teeth are slightly wider, mesial distal, than the mandibular central incisors.
3. The mesioincisal angle is fairly sharp, but the distoincisal angle curves toward the distolingual surface, giving the tooth a twisted appearance when viewed from the incisal aspect.
4. The lingual surface is smooth, without any definite grooves or lines. The mesial and distal marginal ridges are very slight, and the lingual fossa is very shallow.
5. The cingulum on the lingual surface at the cervical third is a very small convexity.
6. When the teeth are viewed from the incisal aspect, more of the distoincisal surface is seen, due to the distolingual curvature of the crown.
7. The contact areas on these teeth differ somewhat from those of the mandibular central incisors in that although the mesial and distal contact areas are in the incisal third, the distal contact area is slightly more cervical.
8. The cervical curvature on the mesial surface is approximately 3 mm and on the distal surface is approximately 2 mm in depth.
9. The roots of these teeth are conical but somewhat broader and flatter on the mesial and the distal surfaces than on the labial or lingual surfaces. Sometimes the roots on these teeth are longer than the roots on the central incisors.

Illustrated below and at the top of the next page are five views of the mandibular right lateral incisor. Study these illustrations and the key points on the preceding page; then take the self-test that follows.

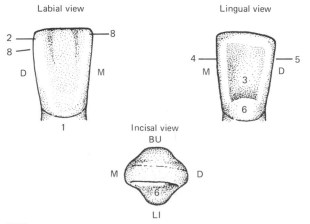

Labial view

Lingual view

Incisal view

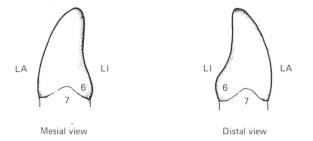

Mesial view   Distal view

Views of the mandibular right lateral incisor. D, distal; M, mesial; LA, labial; LI, lingual. (1) Height of cervical curvature; (2) curvature of distoincisal angle; (3) lingual fossa; (4) mesial marginal ridge; (5) distal marginal ridge; (6) cingulum; (7) cervical curvature; (8) contact area. *Note:* This tooth is larger than the mandibular central incisor.

SELF—TEST

1. The mandibular lateral incisors resemble what other teeth in the dentition? _____

2. Are these teeth larger or smaller than the mandibular central incisors?

_____

3. Describe the appearance of the distoincisal angle. _____

4. From the lingual aspect, does this tooth appear smooth, or does it have a heavy cingulum? _____

5. Do these teeth erupt before the mandibular central incisors? _____

Maxillary Canines: Key Points to Observe

1. The maxillary canines are key teeth. There are two of them, one right and one left. They form the "cornerstones" of the maxillary arch.
2. These are sturdy teeth, well-anchored in the alveolar bone. They mark the transition from anterior teeth to posterior teeth, having some of the features of both the laterals and the first premolars.
3. On the labial surface of the crown, the middle lobe is well developed and normally forms a labial ridge that terminates incisally in a strong cusp or point. On either side of this ridge are shallow developmental depressions.
4. The mesial and distal lobes slope toward the cervical line to form cutting edges or incisal ridges.
5. When observing this tooth from the labial aspect, note the slight concavity on the mesial surface of the crown near the cervical line. All other labial aspects of the crown are well-rounded.
6. On the lingual surface the crown is narrower, with well-developed marginal ridges and a large cingulum.

7. Often there is a lingual ridge extending from the cingulum to the cusp tip, and generally developmental grooves and fossae may be seen on either side.

8. When viewing this tooth from the mesial or distal aspect, note the thickness at the cervical third.

9. The curvature of the cervical line on the mesial surface is 2.5 mm and on the distal surface is 1.5 mm.

10. The contact area on the mesial surface is lower than on the distal.

11. There is one root, the longest of all roots. It is narrow when viewed from the labial or lingual aspect and very broad when viewed from the mesial or distal aspect, tapering at the apex. A shallow groove extends from the cervical line almost to the apex.

Illustrated below are five views of the maxillary right canine. Study these illustrations and the key points on the preceding page; then take the self-test that follows.

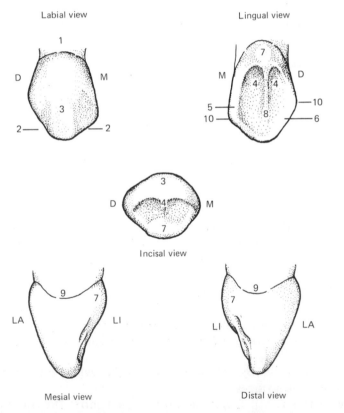

Views of the maxillary right canine. D, distal; M, mesial; LA, labial; LI, lingual. (1) Height of cervical curvature; (2) mesial and distal cutting edges or incisal ridges; (3) labial ridge; (4) lingual fossa; (5) mesial marginal ridge; (6) distal marginal ridge; (7) cingulum; (8) lingual ridge; (9) cervical curvature; (10) contact areas. *Note:* The maxillary and mandibular canines are the longest teeth in the mouth.

1. Is the maxillary canine the third tooth from the median line? _____

2. The function of the canine is: biting; grinding; tearing. (Circle one.)

3. Is the root of the maxillary canine the longest root in the mouth? _____

4. The maxillary canine has one cusp with two distinct cusp ridges. Where are the cusp ridges located? _____

5. Do these teeth form the cornerstones of the maxillary arch? _____

6. Do these teeth have features of both the lateral and the first premolars?
   _____

7. How many lobes form these teeth? _____

8. On the labial surface, which lobe is the most prominent? _____

9. What is this lobe called? _____

10. Do these teeth have a sturdy look? What would be the reason? _____

11. Is the contact area on the mesial surface lower or higher than on the distal surface? _____

12. How many roots are there on these teeth? Are they broad and strong?
    _____

Mandibular Canines: Key Points to Observe

1. The mandibular canines are also "key" teeth. There are two of them, one right and one left. They, like the maxillary canines are the "cornerstones" of their arch—the mandibular arch in this case.

2. These teeth are more slender and more delicate than the maxillary canines, but otherwise resemble them closely.

3. For the labial aspect this tooth is narrower and appears somewhat longer than the maxillary canine. There is a slight concavity in the cervical third on the distal surface, with the mesial surface almost straight.

4. The mesial and distal cutting edges are less pronounced than on the maxillary canines, and the cusp tip is less pointed.

5. There are shallow developmental grooves outlining a shallow labial ridge.

6. The lingual view appears fairly smooth, with the marginal ridges, lingual ridge, fossa, and cingulum much less prominent than on the maxillary canines.

7. The depth of cervical curvature on the mesial surface is 2.5 mm and on the distal surface is 1 mm.

8. The mesial contact area is in the incisal third, and on the distal surface it is near the middle third.

9. The root of this tooth is narrow when viewed from the labial or lingual

aspect. When viewed from the mesial or distal aspect, the root is broader but not so broad as the root of the maxillary canine. There is a shallow depression extending from the cervical line to the apex.

10. Another difference between these teeth and the maxillary canines is that at times there is a bifurcation of the root of the mandibulars, generally occurring in the apical third.

Illustrated below are five views of the mandibular right canine. Study these illustrations and the key points on the preceding page; then take the self-test that follows.

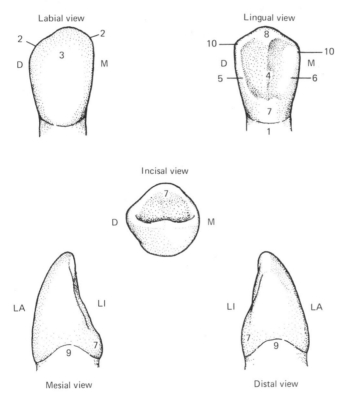

Views of the mandibular right canine. D, distal; M, mesial; LA, labial; LI, lingual. (1) Height of cervical curvature; (2) mesial and distal cutting edges or incisal ridges; (3) labial ridge; (4) lingual fossa; (5) mesial marginal ridge; (6) distal marginal ridge; (7) cingulum; (8) lingual ridge; (9) cervical curvature; (10) contact areas. *Note:* This tooth is much the same as the maxillary canine, but more slender and more delicate.

SELF—TEST

1. Why are the mandibular canine teeth important? _____

2. Are these teeth more slender and delicate than those in the maxillae? _____

3. Do these teeth have a labial ridge? _____

4. In what third is the mesial contact area? The distal contact area? _____

5. How many roots do these teeth have? _____

6. Are these roots bifurcated? _____

7. When viewed from the lingual aspect, are the crowns of these teeth fairly smooth? _____

Maxillary Right First Premolars: Key Points to Observe

1. The maxillary first premolars resemble the canines when observed from the buccal (facial) aspect; however, the crown is shorter and not so wide as that of the canines.
2. From the buccal and lingual view, the crown of this tooth, like that of the canine, is trapezoidal in form, with the narrowest measurement at the cervix and the widest near the occlusal surface. On the buccal surface the middle lobe forms a distinct ridge that terminates on the occlusal surface in a sharp cusp. On either side of this ridge there are shallow depressions. The mesial and distal cutting edges, or cusp ridges, are formed by the shorter and rounder mesial and distal lobes.
3. The contact areas of these teeth are broader than those on the anterior teeth and almost on the same level, rather than at different heights.
4. The height of cervical curvature on the buccal surface is only slightly convex toward the root. It is less than that on the anterior teeth.
5. This tooth is wider from the buccal surface to the lingual surface than it is from the mesial surface to the distal surface, due to the presence of a lingual cusp rather than a cingulum.
6. When observed from the mesial and distal aspect, the crown is trapezoidal in form, but the narrowest measurement is now at the occlusal surface and the widest at the cervix. This is just the opposite of the buccal and lingual view.
7. There is a shallow concavity on the mesial surface of the crown. It is called the *mesial developmental depression*. It extends from just below the contact area to the cervical line, where it joins with a shallow developmental groove on the root. The distal surface is much the same as the mesial surface, but the developmental depression that was noted on the mesial surface is not present.
8. On the occlusal surface a central groove divides the buccal and lingual cusps. Extending from the central groove is a developmental groove that crosses the mesial marginal ridge, just lingual to the mesial contact area.
9. Other features of the occlusal surface are the triangular ridges. One triangular ridge extends from the center of the buccal cusp ridge to the central groove, and one extends from the center of the lingual cusp ridge to the central groove. Together these triangular ridges form a *transverse ridge*.
10. At either end of the central groove, are the mesial and distal triangular

fossae. The mesiobuccal, distobuccal, mesiolingual, and distolingual developmental grooves form part of the boundary of these fossae. Where the peak of the fossa joins the mesial and distal ends of the central groove, there is usually a pit.

11. The depth of cervical curvature on the mesial surface is 1 mm and on the distal surface is 0.5 mm.

12. These teeth generally have two roots that are bifurcated near the apical third. From the buccal or lingual aspect the roots appear narrow, but from the mesial or distal aspect, they are quite wide. On the mesial side of the root, there is a prominent developmental depression extending from cervix to bifurcation. On the distal side of the root this depression is not generally seen. The two roots are situated, one to the buccal and one to the lingual.

Illustrated below are five views of the maxillary right first premolar. Study these illustrations and the key points on the preceding page; then take the self-test that follows.

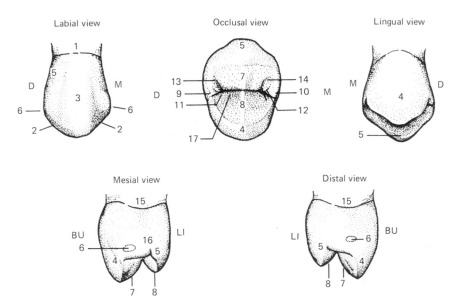

Views of the maxillary right first premolar. D, distal; M, mesial; BU, buccal; LI, lingual. (1) Height of cervical curvature; (2) mesial and distal cusp ridges; (3) buccal ridge; (4) lingual cusp; (5) buccal cusp; (6) contact area; (7) buccal triangular ridge; (8) lingual triangular ridge; (9) distal marginal ridge; (10) mesial marginal ridge; (11) distal triangular fossa; (12) mesial triangular fossa; (13) distobuccal developmental groove; (14) mesiobuccal developmental groove; (15) cervical curvature; (16) mesial developmental groove; (17) central groove. *Note:* Height of cusps. The lingual cusp is 1 mm shorter than the buccal cusp. Both cusps may be seen from the lingual aspect.

SELF—TEST

1. Do the maxillary first premolars resemble the maxillary canines when viewed from the buccal aspect? _____

2. Are there any differences between the maxillary canines and the first premolars? If so, what are they? _____
_____

3. How many lobes form these teeth, and where is the most prominent one? _____

4. Are the contact areas broader than on the anterior teeth? _____

5. Which lobes form the mesial and distal cutting edges on these teeth?
_____

6. Is the height of cervical curvature on the buccal and lingual surfaces of these teeth more rounded or less rounded than that on the anterior teeth? _____

7. What makes these teeth wider from the buccal surface to lingual surface than from mesial surface to distal surface? _____
_____

8. What geometric shape is the crown of the maxillary first premolar when viewed from the buccal aspect? _____

9. What is the shallow concavity called on the mesial surface of the crown? Does it extend to the cervical line and then continue on to the root? Does the distal surface have the same shallow concavity? _____

10. What is the name of the developmental groove that divides the buccal cusp from the lingual cusp? _____

11. What is the name of the developmental groove that crosses over the mesial marginal ridge? _____

12. Where are the triangular ridges on these teeth? Is there a transverse ridge?
_____

13. Where are the fossae, and what are they called? _____
_____

14. Is the depth of the cervical curvature on the mesial and distal surfaces becoming less as the posterior of the arch is approached? _____

15. How many roots do these teeth have? _____

16. Are the roots bifurcated? Trifurcated? If so, in what third does this occur? _____
_____

17. Where are the roots located? _____

185

1. The mandibular first premolars are the first of the posterior teeth in the mandible, and like all of the posterior teeth in the mandible, the buccal surface slopes toward the lingual. When viewed from the mesial or distal aspect, the buccal cusp appears to be almost in the center of the occlusal surface.

2. From the buccal view, the mesial surface and the distal surface are dissimilar. The distal cusp ridge is more convex and much shorter than the mesial cusp ridge, where a definite cusp ridge can be seen. The contact areas, however, are almost at the same height at the junction of the middle and occlusal thirds.

3. There is a ridge extending from the cervical line to the occlusal surface to form a buccal cusp ridge. On either side of this ridge are very slight depressions that mark the joining of the three developmental lobes.

4. From the lingual view most of the buccal cusp can be seen, as the lingual cusp, representing the fourth lobe, is very small.

5. On the occlusal surface, buccal and lingual triangular ridges, forming a transverse ridge, can be seen. The buccal triangular ridge is the largest and strongest.

6. Occasionally there is a central groove; however, it is more often absent.

7. The distal surface of this tooth is much the same as the mesial surface; however, there is no developmental groove crossing the distal marginal ridge, and the contact area is wider than on the mesial.

8. The cervical depth on the mesial surface is 1 mm and on the distal surface is 0.5 mm.

9. When viewed from the occlusal surface, these teeth have a round appearance due to the convexity of the buccal and lingual cusps.

10. As in all posterior teeth, these premolars have a mesial triangular fossa and a distal triangular fossa each formed by the various ridges and grooves that surround them. The peak of the fossa terminates in a pit near the center of the occlusal surface.

11. There is one root that appears narrow from the buccal and lingual aspect. From the mesial and distal aspects, however, the root appears quite broad. There is a developmental depression extending most of the root length, and the apex terminates in a rather sharp point.

12. The contact area on the mesial surface is quite low, and on the distal surface it occurs about midway between the cervical line and the cusp tip.

Five views of the mandibular right first premolar are illustrated on the next page. Study these illustrations and the key points above; then take the self-test that follows.

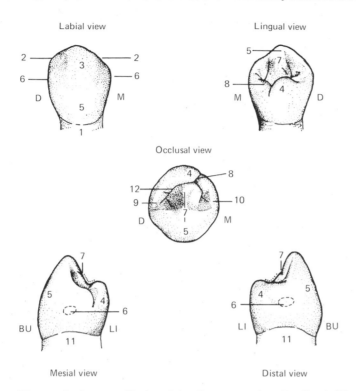

Views of the mandibular right first premolar. D, distal; M, mesial; BU, buccal; LI, lingual. (1) Height of cervical curvature; (2) distal and mesial cusp ridges; (3) buccal ridge; (4) lingual cusp; (5) buccal cusp; (6) contact area; (7) transverse ridge; (8) mesiolingual developmental groove; (9) distal marginal ridge; (10) mesial marginal ridge; (11) cervical curvature; (12) central groove. *Note:* The lingual cusp is very small.

SELF—TEST

1. How many first premolars are there in the mandible? _____

2. Are the contact areas on these teeth almost on the same level when viewed from the buccal aspect? _____

3. How many cusps does the first premolar have? _____

4. Which is the smallest cusp? _____

5. How many roots are there on the first premolar? _____

6. Are there triangular ridges on the occlusal surface? If so, which one is more prominent? _____
_____

7. Is there a mesiolingual groove on these teeth? _____

8. When observed from the mesial aspect, does the crown tip toward the lingual or toward the buccal? _____

9. How many roots do these teeth have? _____

10. Is the cervical curvature on the mesial surface greater or lesser than on the distal surface? _____

Maxillary Second Premolars: Key Points to Observe

1. The maxillary second premolars are similar to the maxillary first premolars; however, they are more round. When viewed from the buccal (facial) aspect, the buccal cusp is not as pointed as the cusp on the first premolar; also the mesial cusp ridge is shorter than the distal cusp ridge.
2. The buccal cusp and the lingual cusp are almost equal in length.
3. When viewed from the occlusal surface, this tooth appears wider than the maxillary first premolar, from the buccal cusp ridge to the lingual cusp ridge, thus giving the teeth a wide-open appearance.
4. There are strong, well-rounded mesial and distal marginal ridges, on the occulusal surface.
5. There is a triangular ridge extending from the tip of the buccal cusp and the lingual cusp to the central groove. These ridges, although not as prominent as the triangular ridges on the maxillary first premolars, do form a transverse ridge.
6. One of the main differences that distinguishes this tooth from the maxillary first premolar is the short central groove on the occlusal surface. There are many supplementary grooves radiating from this central groove toward the buccal and the lingual surfaces, giving the occlusal surface a wrinkled appearance.
7. The depth of cervical curvature is the same as on the first premolar.
8. There is one root that is narrow when viewed from the buccal aspect. When viewed from the mesial or distal aspects the root is broad. There are shallow developmental grooves extending from the cervix to the apex. When viewed from the lingual aspect much of the buccal surface of the root shows, due to the narrowness of the lingual surface.

Illustrated below and on the next page are five views of the maxillary right second premolar. Study these illustrations and the key points above and then take the self-test that follows.

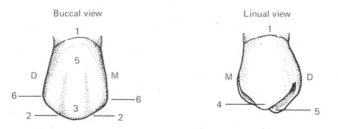

Buccal view   Linual view

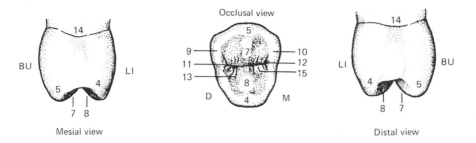

Views of the maxillary right second premolar. D, distal; M, mesial; BU, buccal; LI, lingual. (1) Height of cervical curvature; (2) mesial and distal cusp ridges; (3) buccal ridge; (4) lingual cusp; (5) buccal cusp; (6) contact area; (7) buccal triangular ridge; (8) lingual triangular ridge; (9) distal marginal ridge; (10) mesial marginal ridge; (11) distal triangular fossa; (12) mesial triangular fossa; (13) supplementary grooves; (14) cervical curvature; (15) central groove.

SELF—TEST

1. The maxillary second premolars are similar to the first premolars, but there are three differences. Name these differences. _____

_____

2. Are there two cusps, and are they equal in length? _____

3. From the occlusal view, are these teeth wider than the maxillary first premolars, from the buccal cusp ridge to the lingual cusp ridge? _____

4. Where are the marginal ridges? _____

5. Are there triangular ridges on the occlusal surface? If so, where are they located, and do they or do they not form a transverse ridge? _____

_____

6. What gives these teeth a wrinkled appearance? _____

7. How many roots are there? Is the root, or roots, narrower buccolingually or mesiodistally? _____

_____

Mandibular Second Premolars: Key Points to Observe

1. When viewed from the buccal aspect, the mandibular second premolars are similar to the mandibular first premolars. However, they are slightly larger, and the buccal cusp is shorter than the buccal cusp on the first premolar.
2. There is a fairly well-developed buccal ridge on the buccal surface, with shallow developmental grooves on either side.

3. The mesial and distal cusp ridges are short and less angled than on the first premolar, giving these teeth a round appearance from the buccal aspect.

4. On the lingual surface there are two cusps that are slightly shorter than the buccal cusp.

5. When viewed from the occlusal aspect, the crown appears trapezoidal, with the widest part on the buccal side and the narrowest part on the lingual side.

6. The mesial and distal marginal ridges are well-rounded, and the mesial and distal triangular fossae on either end of a fairly short central groove are fairly distinct.

7. Dividing the two lingual cusps is the lingual developmental groove, which, together with the central groove and the mesiobuccal and distobuccal developmental grooves, forms a "Y" configuration. There is a central pit where these developmental grooves meet.

8. There are three triangular ridges on the occlusal surface. One triangular ridge extends from the buccal cusp ridge to the central groove, and one extends from the distolingual cusp ridge to the central groove. The third triangular ridge extends from the mesiolingual cusp ridge to the central groove.

9. The contact areas are broad. They are located in the occlusal third of the crown.

10. The curvature at the cervical line is very slight, no more than 1 mm.

11. These teeth have one root that is wider buccolingually than mesio-distally. It is a fairly flat root. At times there is a shallow developmental groove extending on the mesial surface from the middle third to the apex.

Illustrated below and on the next page are five views of the mandibular right second premolar. Study these illustrations and the key points on the preceding page; then take the self-test that follows.

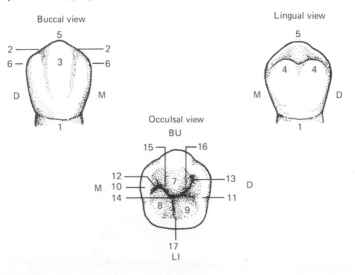

Buccal view

Lingual view

Occulsal view

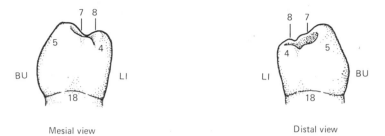

Mesial view   Distal view

Views of the mandibular right second premolar. D, distal; M, mesial; BU, buccal; LI, lingual. (1) Height of cervical curvature; (2) mesial and distal cusp ridges; (3) buccal ridge; (4) lingual cusps; (5) buccal cusp; (6) contact area; (7) buccal triangular ridge; (8) lingual triangular ridge, mesial; (9) lingual triangular ridge, distal; (10) mesial marginal ridge; (11) distal marginal ridge; (12) mesial triangular fossa; (13) distal triangular fossa; (14) central pit; (15) mesial developmental groove; (16) distal developmental groove; (17) lingual developmental groove; (18) cervical curvature.

SELF—TEST

1. Are the mandibular second premolars similar to the first mandibular premolars, when viewed from the buccal aspect? _____

2. Do these teeth appear more round from the buccal aspect? _____

3. How many cusps do these teeth have, and where are they located? _____

_____

4. What configuration appears most frequently on the occlusal surface, as a result of the placement of the central groove and the mesiobuccal and distobuccal developmental grooves? _____

5. How many triangular ridges are there on the occlusal surface? _____

6. Are the contact areas broad or narrow? _____

7. Give the location of the contact areas on the crown. _____

Maxillary First Molars: Key Points to Observe

1. The maxillary first molars are the largest and strongest teeth in the maxillary arch.

2. They have four major cusps, three of which are well developed, with one smaller cusp. Two of the well-developed cusps are on the buccal side, the mesiobuccal cusp and the distobuccal cusp, and the other two are on the lingual side, with the distolingual cusp the smallest of the four cusps, and the mesiolingual cusp the largest of the four cusps. The small or supplemental cusp is sometimes called the *cusp of Carabelli*. It is located on the mesiolingual cusp 2 to 3 mm below the occlusal surface. Generally this cusp is of little importance. However, it may be prominent, giving the lingual surface, when viewed from the mesial or distal aspect, greater convexity at that point.

3. The crown of these teeth, when observed from the buccal or the lingual aspect, is roughly trapezoidal in form. From the buccal view, parts of all four cusps may be seen, with the mesiolingual cusp the most prominent. It can be seen between the mesiobuccal and the distobuccal cusps. Part of the distolingual cusp may be seen to the distal side of the distobuccal cusp, due to the rhomboidal form of the occlusal surface. From the lingual aspect the tooth is quite different, as the buccal cusps do not show; and only the large mesiolingual cusp and the small, rounded distolingual cusp can be seen.

4. The mesial surface from the buccal and lingual views is fairly straight from the cervix to the contact area in the occlusal third. The distal surface is quite convex.

5. The buccal and the lingual developmental grooves that divide the two buccal cusps and the two lingual cusps are quite prominent, extending at times, well into the middle third of the buccal and lingual surfaces of the crown.

6. When viewed from the mesial or distal aspect, the crown is wider than when viewed from the buccal or lingual aspect; however, it is still roughly trapezoidal in form. The buccal outline of the crown, when viewed from the mesial and distal aspect, is slightly convex, just above the cervical line; it then tapers toward the occlusal surface and the tips of the mesiobuccal and distobuccal cusps. The lingual outline is much the same as the buccal outline, but the convexity is higher; it is in the middle third. If the fifth cusp is outstanding, the lingual outline is quite different in that the developmental groove outlining the cusp is deeper, and the height of curvature is more pronounced.

7. The mesial marginal ridge and the distal marginal ridge are on the occlusal surface, joining the mesiobuccal cusp ridge to the mesiolingual cusp ridge, and the distobuccal cusp ridge to the distolingual cusp ridge. About midway between the cusps the marginal ridges dip toward the cervical line. The depth of curvature of these ridges is greater on the distal side than on the mesial side allowing the triangular ridges to be seen from the distal aspect. The cervical line, from both views, shows some depth toward the occlusal but not more than 0.5 mm to 1 mm. The greater depth is on the mesial surface.

8. When viewed from the occlusal surface, the crown appears to be somewhat rhomboidal.

9. There is a well-developed oblique ridge transversing the occlusal surface in an oblique fashion from the distobuccal cusp to the mesiolingual cusp. This ridge is the approximate height of the marginal ridges, as it dips down from the distobuccal cusp and mesiolingual cusp. At times, a developmental groove may divide the buccal portion of the oblique ridge from the lingual portion. This oblique ridge is found to some extent on all maxillary molars, but it is most prominent on the maxillary first molar.

10. There are two major fossae on the occlusal surface, the central and the distal fossae. The central fossa is a depression, just mesial to the oblique ridge. It is somewhat concave, ending in the central developmental pit on the occlusal surface. The distal fossa is just distal to the oblique ridge. Both fossae are formed by the slopes, the cusps, the oblique ridge, and the triangular ridges in that area.

11. There are two minor triangular fossae, the mesial triangular fossa and the distal triangular fossa. They are located either mesial or distal to their respective marginal ridges. The base of the mesial triangular fossa is toward the mesial marginal ridge, and the apex occurs where supplemental grooves join the central groove. The distal triangular fossa is just distal to the oblique ridge, with its base toward the distal marginal ridge and the apex at the distal developmental oblique groove.

12. The buccal developmental groove that divides the two buccal cusps extends to the buccal surface from the central developmental pit.

13. The central developmental groove extends toward the mesial from the central pit. This groove extends toward the mesial triangular fossa, where supplemenal grooves extend from it to outline the fossa.

14. On the distal side of the occlusal surface can be seen the distal oblique groove, extending along the distal side of the oblique ridge and then connecting with the lingual groove that divides the mesiolingual and distolingual cusps.

15. From the mesial aspect of these triple-rooted teeth only the lingual and mesiobuccal roots can be seen. From the distal and the buccal aspects all three roots can be seen with the lingual (palatal) root the longest and the distobuccal root the shortest.

Illustrated below and on the next page are five views of the maxillary right first molar. Study these illustrations and the key points on the preceding page; then take the self-test that follows.

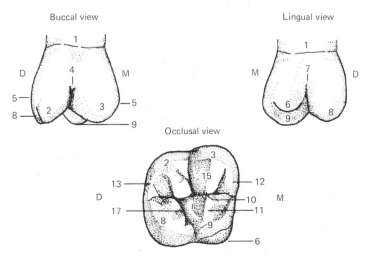

Buccal view

Lingual view

Occlusal view

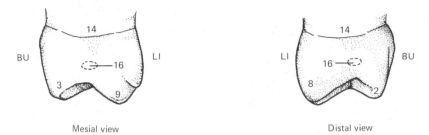

Mesial view   Distal view

Views of the maxillary right first molar. D, distal; M, mesial; BU, buccal; LI, lingual. (1) Cervical line; (2) distobuccal cusp; (3) mesiobuccal cusp; (4) buccal groove; (5) crest of curvature; (6) cusp of Carabelli; (7) distolingual groove; (8) distolingual cusp; (9) mesiolingual cusp; (10) central groove; (11) oblique ridge; (12) mesial marginal ridge; (13) distal marginal ridge; (14) cervical curvature; (15) buccal triangular ridge; (16) contact area; (17) distal developmental groove.

SELF—TEST

1. How many cusps do the maxillary first molars have? _____

2. Where are they located? Name them. _____

3. What is the cusp of Carabelli? Where is it located? _____

4. Do the lingual cusps show when these teeth are viewed from the buccal aspect? _____

5. Which is the largest cusp? _____

6. Which is the smallest of the major cusps? _____

7. Name the developmental grooves that divide the cusps. _____

8. What gometric shape does the crown assume when viewed from the occlusal surface? _____

9. Where is the oblique ridge? From what cusp to what cusp does it extend?

_____

10. Name the two major fossae on the occlusal surface. _____

11. Name the two minor triangular fossae, and give their location. _____

_____

12. Locate the buccal pit and the central pit. _____

13. How many roots do these teeth have? Where are they located? _____

_____

Mandibular Right First Molars: Key Points to Observe

1. The mandibular first molars are generally the largest and strongest teeth in the mandibular arch.

2. The crown has five cusps, four major cusps, and one smaller cusp. Two of the major cusps are on the buccal side of the crown and two on the lingual side, with the smaller cusp on the distal side. All five cusps can be seen from the buccal aspect because the lingual cusps are higher than the buccal cusps and more pointed. The small distal cusp is quite convex in the occlusal third.

3. There are two developmental grooves on the buccal surface of the crown, the mesiobuccal developmental groove and the distobuccal developmental groove. The mesiobuccal developmental groove separates the mesiobuccal cusp from the distobuccal cusp, and the distobuccal developmental groove separates the distobuccal cusp from the distal cusp. On the lingual surface there is only one developmental groove, the lingual developmental groove; it separates the mesiolingual cusp from the distolingual cusp.

4. The crown, when viewed from the buccal or lingual aspect, is roughly trapezoidal.

5. When viewed from the occlusal aspect, the crown of these teeth is wider from mesial to distal than from buccal to lingual. The crown narrows toward the lingual surface.

6. When viewed from the mesial or distal aspect, the buccal surface of the crown shows a marked convexity in the cervical third; it then slopes gently toward the lingual surface. The lingual surface is rounder than the buccal surface, with a slight concavity rather than convexity in the cervical third. The crown of this tooth is shorter on the distal surface than on the mesial surface from the occlusal surface to the cervical line, thus exposing a portion of the occlusal surface. The distobuccal developmental groove can also be seen from this view. From the mesial aspect only the mesiobuccal cusp, mesial marginal ridge, and the mesiolingual cusp can be seen.

7. On the mesial and distal surfaces the cervical line is irregular. It dips toward the root on the mesial surface and 0.5 mm on the distal surface.

8. When viewed from the occlusal aspect, the buccal and lingual surfaces are convex.

9. A central groove divides the buccal cusps from the lingual cusps as it travels across the occlusal surface from mesial to distal.

10. There is one major fossa on the occlusal surface: the central fossa from which extend the mesiobuccal developmental groove, the distobuccal developmental groove, and the lingual developmental groove. All of these grooves terminate in a pit in the center of the central fossa. This pit is called the *central pit*.

11. There are two minor triangular fossae, the mesial triangular fossa and the distal triangular fossa, the mesial triangular fossa being the more distinct. Each has its base at the corresponding marginal ridge and its apex terminating in a pit at either end of the central groove.

12. There are several triangular ridges descending from the cusp tips to the central fossa. They descend from the mesiobuccal cusp to the mesio-

lingual cusp, forming a transverse ridge, and from the distobuccal cusp to the distolingual cusp to form another transverse ridge. The triangular ridge on the distal cusp does not meet another triangular ridge but extends down to the central groove, where it terminates.

13. Many supplemental grooves may be seen on the occlusal surface.

14. These teeth have two roots, one mesial and one distal. The roots are much wider when viewed from the mesial or distal aspect than when viewed from the buccal or lingual aspect. The bifurcation occurs where the cervical third and the middle third meet. The mesial root has a deep depression running from the cervical line to the blunt apex. Within the mesial root are two canals, the mesiobuccal canal and the distobuccal canal. The distal root has only one canal.

Illustrated below are five views of the mandibular right first molar. Study these illustrations and the key points on the preceding page, and then take the self-test that follows.

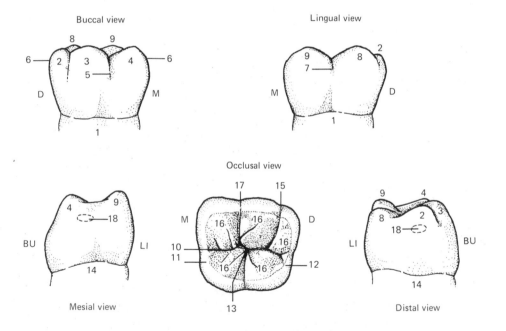

Views of the mandibular right first molar. D, distal; M, mesial; BU, buccal; LI, lingual. (1) Cervical line; (2) distal cusp; (3) distobuccal cusp; (4) mesiobuccal cusp; (5) mesiobuccal developmental groove; (6) crest of curvature; (7) lingual developmental groove; (8) distolingual cusp; (9) mesiolingual cusp; (10) central groove; (11) mesial marginal ridge; (12) distal marginal ridge; (13) central pit; (14) cervical curvature; (15) distobuccal developmental groove; (16) triangular ridges; (17) buccal developmental groove; (18) contact area.

1. How many cusps do the mandibular first molars have? Name them.
   _____

2. What cusps can be seen from the buccal aspect? _____

3. Are the lingual cusps higher than the buccal cusps? _____

4. When viewed from the occlusal aspect, is the crown of these teeth wider from buccal to lingual or from mesial to distal? _____

5. Beginning in the middle third and extending to the occlusal surface, will the crown of these teeth slope toward the lingual surface? _____

6. Name the groove that divides the buccal cusps from the lingual cusps.
   _____

7. The mesiobuccal developmental groove and the distobuccal developmental groove with the lingual developmental groove form a fossa. What is this fossa called? _____

8. There are fossae and developmental grooves on the occlusal surface of these teeth that terminate in a pit. Name them and tell where they terminate. _____
   _____

9. Are there many triangular ridges on the occlusal surface? Do any form transverse ridges? _____

10. How many roots do these teeth have? Locate them. _____

11. Is there more than one canal in any of the roots? If so, which one or ones? _____

Maxillary Right Second and Third Molars: Key Points to Observe

1. The maxillary second molars are similar in appearance to the maxillary first molars: however, they are smaller, and there are only four cusps on the crown. The cusps are the mesiobuccal, distobuccal, mesiolingual, and distolingual. The distolingual cusp is smaller than that on the maxillary first molar.
2. From the mesial and distal views, the second molar is much the same as the maxillary first molar.
3. The occlusal surface is also very similar to that of the maxillary first molar, but the oblique ridge is not as pronounced, and there are more supplemental grooves.
4. The cervical line is irregular and curves only slightly toward the occlusal surface.

5. There are three roots, but they are not as widespread as on the maxillary first molar.
6. The maxillary third molars are similar to the maxillary second molars, but they too are generally smaller.
7. The distolingual cusp on the maxillary third molar is very small and sometimes is missing altogether.
8. The maxillary third molars are frequently deformed or missing altogether.
9. The roots on the maxillary third molars vary in number and many times are fused together.

Illustrated below are five views of the maxillary right second molar. The third molar will not be shown. Study these illustrations and the key points on the preceding page; then take the self-test that follows.

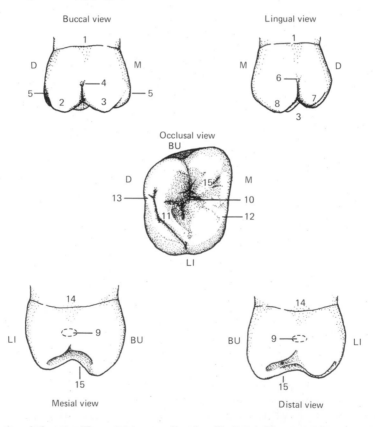

Views of the maxillary right second molar. D, distal; M, mesial; BU, buccal; LI, lingual. (1) Cervical line; (2) distobuccal cusp; (3) mesiobuccal cusp; (4) buccal groove; (5) crest of curvature; (6) distolingual groove; (7) distolingual cusp; (8) mesiolingual cusp; (9) contact area; (10) central groove; (11) oblique ridge; (12) mesial marginal ridge; (13) distal marginal ridge; (14) cervical curvature; (15) buccal triangular ridge. *Note:* There is no cusp of Carabelli on these molars.

1. How many cusps are there on the maxillary second molar? Which cusp is the smallest? _____

2. Are the maxillary second molars larger or smaller than the maxillary first molars? _____

3. Does this tooth have the same occlusal anatomy as the maxillary first molar? _____

4. How many roots are there on the maxillary second molar? Name them.

_____

5. Are the maxillary third molars larger or smaller than the maxillary second molars? _____

6. Is the distal cusp on the maxillary third molar larger or smaller than the distal cusp on the maxillary first molar? _____

7. Are the maxillary third molars sometimes deformed or missing? _____

8. Are the roots of the maxillary third molars sometimes fused? _____

9. How many roots are there on the maxillary third molar? _____

Mandibular Right Second and Third Molars: Key Points to Observe

1. The mandibular second molars are generally smaller than the mandibular first molars.
2. There are four cusps of equal size, with the distobuccal cusp larger than that on the first molar, apparently to compensate for the absence of the distal cusp on these teeth.
3. The four cusps are divided almost equally by a central groove that extends across the occlusal surface from mesial to distal, with a triangular fossa at either end, a buccal developmental groove that extends from the central groove to the buccal, and a lingual developmental groove that extends from the central groove to the lingual surface.
4. The tips of the lingual cusps can be seen from the buccal aspect, just as they can on the first molars.
5. The mesial and distal outlines are very similar to those of the first molars, with the exception of the distal cusp and the distobuccal developmental groove, which are absent on these teeth.
6. There are two roots, one mesial and one distal. These roots tend to lean toward the distal more than do the roots on the first molars.
7. The mandibular third molars are generally so varied a true description is very difficult.
8. In general, the mandibular third molars are similar to the mandibular second molars from all views. They do, however, tend to be larger.

9. There are two roots on these teeth, but multirooted teeth are not unknown.

Illustrated below are five views of the mandibular right second molar. The third molar will not be shown. Study these illustrations and the key points on the preceding page; then take the self-test that follows.

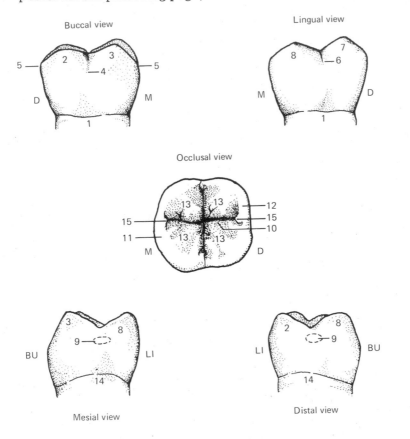

Views of the mandibular right second molar. D, digital; M, mesial; BU, buccal; LI, lingual. (1) Cervical line; (2) distobuccal cusp; (3) mesiobuccal cusp; (4) buccal groove; (5) crest of curvature; (6) distolingual groove; (7) distolingual cusp; (8) mesiolingual cusp; (9) contact area; (10) central groove; (11) mesial marginal ridge; (12) distal marginal ridge; (13) triangular ridges; (14) cervical curvature; (15) mesial and distal fossae.

SELF—TEST

1. How many cusps are there on the mandibular second molar? Name them.

2. Are the cusps divided almost equally by the developmental grooves?

3. Is there a distal cusp on the mandibular second molar? _____

4. Are the lingual cusps on the mandibular second molar higher than those on the buccal cusps? _____

5. How many roots are there on the mandibular second molar? Name them.

_____

6. Do the mandibular third molars tend to be larger than the mandibular second molars? _____

7. How many roots are there on the mandibular third molars? _____

8. Are there always the same number of roots on the mandibular third molars? _____

9. Why are these third molars difficult to describe accurately? _____

CARVING THE TEETH

How to Use the Boley Gauge

When it is necessary to measure any part of a tooth, a Vernier-type instrument is very useful. The Vernier scale (movable jaw) on the Boley gauge is used for measuring in the metric system. It was devised by Pierre Vernier, a French mathematician. It is so constructed that one can easily measure a part of a tooth to within one-tenth (0.1) of a millimeter (mm). However, for this exercise, only units of whole millimeters and half (0.5) millimeters will be used.

The bar of the Boley gauge is divided into ten equal spaces. Each space is 9 mm in length. The total bar length is 100 mm. The Boley gauge consists of three major parts: the base jaw, the bar scale, and the movable jaw. The movable jaw has ten 1-mm spaces that are not numbered. The first line on both the bar scale and the slide scale is the index line. When the zero division on the main scale and the index line on the movable jaw are together, the instrument does not register any measurement. To measure in millimeters, place the thumb in the notch on the Vernier scale and pull or push the movable jaw along the bar scale. To lock the Vernier scale in place, pull on the lock lever with the index finger.

The Boley gauge is used to measure undercut parts of a tooth, and to measure widths or lengths. Use the curved jaws for measuring undercuts, and use the straight jaws to measure widths or lengths.

There are two sets of numbers on the bar scale. The lower set of numbers is the one you will use for this exercise because it indicates the distance between the jaws. The upper set of numbers, which is inverted, is used as a depth gauge. (See the illustration on the next page.)

To read the Vernier scale (sliding scale), move the index line to the right, exactly halfway between the second and third short lines after the "2." The window would look like the illustration on the next page. This would give you a reading of 22.5 mm.

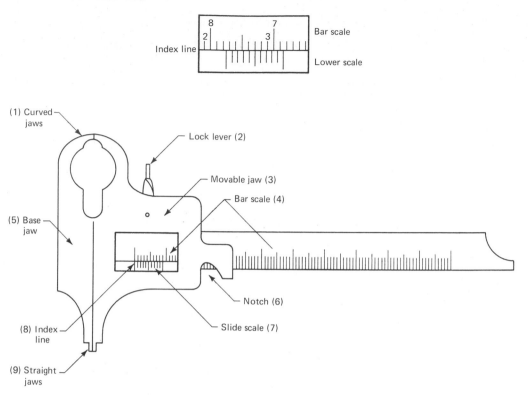

The Boley gauge. (1) Curved jaws; (2) lock lever; (3) movable jaw; (4) bar scale; (5) base jaw; (6) notch; (7) slide scale; (8) index line; (9) straight jaws.

SELF—TEST

1. Why is a Boley gauge used? _____

2. What is the smallest measurement made with this instrument? _____

3. Name the major parts. _____

4. When is the curved jaw used? _____

5. When is the straight jaw used? _____

6. Open the Boley gauge so that the index line appears as illustrated below. When the index line is on the long line to the right of the "1," the jaws are exactly how far apart? _____

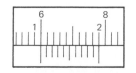

7. Close the jaws until the index line is on the long line that is halfway between the "0" and the "1." What is the reading? _____

8. Now open the jaws so that the index line is on the long line in between the "2" and "3." What is the reading? _____

9. Next close the jaws until the index line is on the third short line after the "2." What is the reading now? _____

Carving the Teeth from Wax Cubes

Instruments and Materials Required

1. Study wax cubes
2. Boley gauge
3. Millimeter rule (plastic)
4. Laboratory knife
5. ½ Hollenback carver
6. Cleoid-discoid carver
7. Wax spatula #7
8. Bunsen burner
9. Matches
10. Container for wax scraps
11. Illustrations of tooth anatomy

Tooth to be Carved: Maxillary First Premolar

Steps in Carving

I. Measuring and marking the wax cube. (See illustrations below.)

A. Using the #7 wax spatula or the cleoid, carve the letters BU for "buccal." Turn the cube over and place the letters LI on the other side for "lingual."

B. Find the center of the long axis of the cube by using the mm rule to measure the width. The center line should be about 6.5 mm from each side, as each block of wax is approximately 13 mm wide.

C. Draw a line down through the center of the cube both on the buccal and lingual sides.

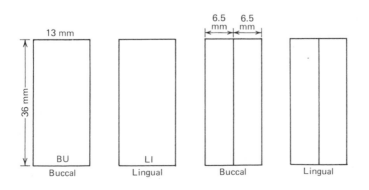

II. Establishing the length of the crown. (See figures below.)

    A. Measure 3 mm down, on the buccal side. Draw a line across the cube at that point and place the letters OC (occlusal) in this area.

    B. Do the same on the lingual side.

    C. Using the tooth measurement guide, establish the length of the crown by measuring 8.5 mm down from the last established line.

    D. Draw a line across the width of the cube at this point, both on the buccal and the lingual sides.

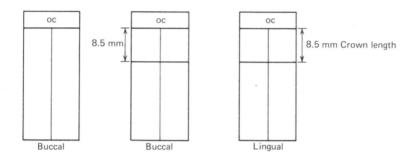

III. Establishing the length of the root.

    A. To establish the length of the root, measure down 14 mm from the last established line that marked the length of crown.

    B. Draw a line at this point across the cube on both the buccal and lingual sides, as shown below.

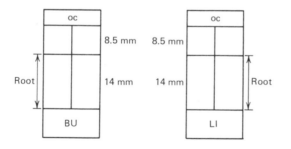

IV. Establishing the mesial-distal width of the crown at the occlusal surface and cervical line.

    A. To establish the width of the crown, measure down about 3 mm from the line marking the occlusal surface. This will be the widest part of the crown from mesial to distal on this tooth.

    B. Place one mark on either side of the center line to establish the width, which is 7 mm. There will be 3.5 mm on either side.

    C. To establish the width of the crown at the cervix, measure 5 mm at the point where the crown and the root meet. This will allow about 2.5 mm on either side of the center line.

    D. Do the same on the lingual side.

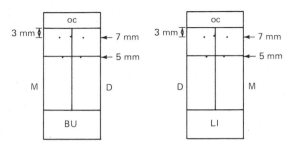

V. Drawing the buccal and lingual outlines of the maxillary first pre-
    molar.
    A. Observe the following buccal and lingual illustrations of the maxil-
       lary first premolar. Using the illustrations as a guide, try to establish
       the outline in your mind.
    B. Draw in the buccal and lingual views of both the crown and root
       by following the illustrations below and the marks previously
       established on the cube. Use the cleoid.

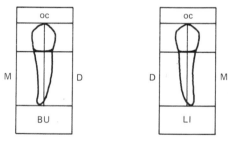

VI. Wax removal from the distal and the mesial surfaces of the cube.
     A. Using the lab knife, carefully remove all of the wax from the
        distal and the mesial surfaces to within 1 mm of the outlines
        drawn on the buccal and lingual surfaces.
     B. Be very careful not to go closer than 1 mm to the drawing. This
        excess wax will be removed later.
     C. Be certain that the buccal and the lingual surfaces are the same.
     D. Be certain that the distal and mesial surfaces are smooth and even.
     E. After removing the wax from the mesial and distal surfaces, your
        wax cube should look like this from the buccal aspect.

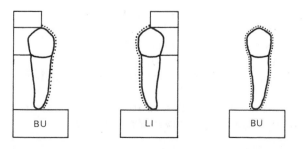

VII. Establishing the measurements on the mesial and the distal surfaces.
   A. Reestablish all measurements now on the mesial and the distal surfaces and label the surfaces.
   B. On the mesial side measure for the width of the crown, which is about 2 mm below the cervical line. The width of the crown will be about 9 mm or 4.5 mm on either side of the center line.
   C. Measure and mark the width at the cervix. This measurement will be approximately 8 mm, or 4 mm on either side of the center line. Do the same on the distal side. Cube will look like this from the buccomesial aspect.

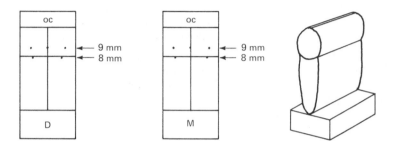

VIII. Drawing in the mesial and distal views of the maxillary first premolar.
   A. Using the cleoid, draw in the mesial and distal views, using the illustrations below as your guide.
   B. Note that the cervix curves slightly toward the occlusal surface, about 1 mm on the mesial side, and so little on the distal side that it isn't worth measuring.

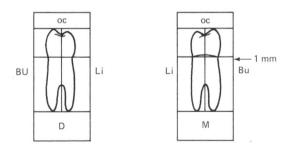

IX. Wax removal from the buccal and the lingual surfaces.
   A. Using the lab knife, remove all of the wax from the buccal and the lingual surfaces down to within 1 mm of the drawing.
   B. Be careful to do this slowly and smoothly.
   C. Remove excess wax on the occlusal surface to within 1 mm of the drawing.
   D. Carve the wax from between the roots. Be very careful not to break them. The ½ Hollenback carver is good to use.

E. Carve the sulcus on the occlusal surface. It will be about 1 mm in depth. After you remove the wax from the buccal and lingual surfaces, your wax cube should look something like this from the distal side.

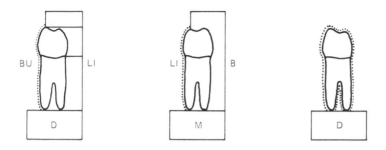

X.   Reestablishing crown and root length; reestablishing crown and cervical width.

A. Use the Boley gauge and remeasure the crown and the root.

B. Do this from the buccal, lingual, mesial, and distal sides.

C. Using the Boley gauge, reestablish the crown width and the cervical width of the labial, lingual, mesial, and distal sides.

XI.   Finishing and Polishing

A. Beginning with the root, continue to shape it by using the Hollenback carver. Be careful not to break it from the stand. Go slowly. It is much easier to remove wax than to add it on. If you should remove too much wax and find that you must add on, melt some of the wax shavings in the Bunsen burner flame, being careful not to overheat the wax. Add it in small amounts until the measurements are correct.

B. After completion of the root, shape the crown, using the Hollenback carver and the cleoid. Measure often.

C. To carve the occlusal surface, establish the width between cusps, which will be about 6 mm. Then cut the inclined planes, both buccal and lingual, that lead up to the triangular ridges.

D. Establish the central groove and the mesiobuccal and distobuccal developmental grooves, marginal ridges, and the triangular fossa. Complete any other details.

E. When the wax tooth has been completed, use a gauze sponge or a small piece of silk, or any other fine smooth cloth, and rub the wax gently until it has a high shine.

All the other teeth may be carved using these directions, the correct tooth measurements, and the illustrations for each tooth. The occlusal surface of the posterior teeth is the most important surface for the dental auxiliary. It is suggested that after the first tooth has been completed for practice, only the crowns of the other posterior teeth need to be carved.

Tooth Measurement Guide for Tooth Carving

Tooth	Root Lengths		Crown Length	Mesiodistal Crown-Cervix Width		Labiolingual Crown-Cervix Width		Cervical Curvature Mesial/Distal	
Maxillae									
Central		13 mm	10.5	8.0	6.5	7.5	6.5	3.5	2.5
Lateral		13 mm	9.0	6.5	5.0	6.5	5.5	3.0	2.0
Canine		16 mm	10.0	7.5	5.5	8.0	7.0	2.5	1.5
1st Premolar		14 mm	8.5	7.0	5.0	9.0	8.0	1.0	0.5
2nd Premolar		14 mm	8.5	6.5	4.5	8.8	7.8	1.0	0.5
1st Molar	LI	13 mm							
	MB	12 mm	7.5	9.5	7.5	11.0	10.0	1.0	0.5
	DB	10 mm							
2nd Molar	LI	12 mm							
	MB	11 mm	7.0	9.0	6.5	10.7	9.8	1.0	0.5
	DB	10 mm							
Mandible									
Central		12.5 mm	9.0	5.0	3.5	6.5	6.0	3.0	2.0
Lateral		14.0 mm	9.5	5.5	4.0	7.0	6.2	3.0	2.0
Canine		16.0 mm	11.0	6.5	5.0	8.0	7.3	2.5	1.0
1st Premolar		14.0 mm	8.5	7.0	5.0	7.5	6.5	1.0	0.5
2nd Premolar		14.5 mm	8.5	7.0	5.0	8.0	7.0	1.0	0.5
1st Molar		14.0 mm	7.5	10.5	8.5	10.0	8.5	1.0	0.5
2nd Molar		13.0 mm	7.0	10.0	7.5	9.5	8.0	1.0	0.5

LI, lingual; MB, mesiobuccal; DB, distobuccal.

5

Microorganisms and Sterilization

HISTORY

Microbiology is the fascinating study of minute one-celled plants and animals, so small that one hundred, side by side, would be no larger than a grain of sand. The study of this logical science is essential to persons involved in any of the health professions, for they must understand the causes and the order of disease transfer, as well as the precautions necessary to prevent such transfer.

These minute bits of life can be seen only through a microscope. Although small, the microorganisms are powerful; those that are harmful can be disastrous to the human animal as war can be. Fortunately, not all microorganisms are harmful. Many contribute to our well-being and some, the body's normal flora, are necessary for our very survival.

As early as the thirteenth century an astute scientist suspected, but was not able to prove, that disease was produced by invisible living creatures. By the early 1600s microscopes were in use, but it wasn't until the latter part of the seventeenth century (1675) that a Dutch dry goods merchant, Anton van Leeuwenhoek (La′-ven-ho͞ok) (1632-1723), often called the "Father of Microbiology," made the first known high-powered microscope with such a well-ground lens that living minute plants and animals could be examined in detail. Van Leeuwenhoek examined rainwater, tartar from his teeth, and many other substances, and much to his amazement, discovered tiny creatures of many shapes and sizes, some of which moved rapidly. He reported his observations, but not the secret of how he ground the high-powered lens, to the Royal Society of London. His data generated renewed interest in the origin of living things, an interest, however, only in the most minute bits of life as they related to higher forms, for the theory of spontaneous generation (the generation of life from nonliving matter) was still believed to be true.

When van Leeuwenhoek died, he took the secret of grinding a high-powered lens with him. This slowed the study of microorganisms, and for many years the battle waged between scientists who believed all living things sprang from nonliving matter and those who did not. The believers in spontaneous generation cited the fact that when meat was exposed to warmth and air, it decayed; and maggots, or life in another form, appeared. The opponents of spontaneous generation believed that life could originate only by the reproduction of life from living organisms. They believed that airborne microorganisms were actually the cause of maggots appearing in meat. They did not believe that maggots appeared spontaneously as a result of putrefaction (rotting).

In the early seventeenth century, poet-physician Francesco Redi (1626-1697) experimented by placing meat in a jar and covering it with gauze. Flies were attracted to the meat, laid their eggs on the gauze, and eventually maggots developed. Although it would seem this would prove maggots did not develop spontaneously from the decaying meat but from something that was airborne, there was still much doubt, and the battle continued between those who believed in spontaneous generation and those who did not.

In 1765, almost a century later, Lazzaro Spallanzani an Italian biologist, (1729-1799), performed many experiments in his attempt to disprove spontaneous generation. In one of these experiments he boiled beef broth in a flask from which all air had been removed. The flask was then hermetically sealed. Upon examination of the broth, he found no microbes. This should have settled the argument of spontaneous generation, but it did not. Some of the doubters still believed that eels originated from mud, and mice from cheese, or maggots from putrified meat; for during early experiments, scientists did not observe the same precautions Spallanzani took, and they permitted air to contaminate their experiments.

It wasn't until Louis Pasteur, a professor of chemistry (1822-1895), irritated by some of the faulty logic and data being presented, performed the experiments (1861-1864) that finally settled the argument of spontaneous generation. Through well-controlled experiments Pasteur proved beyond a doubt that airborne bacteria were the cause of some disease. This discovery is known as the "Germ Theory of Disease," beginning what is sometimes called the "Golden Age of Microbiology" (1880-1910).

Before the time of Pasteur's proof that airborne microorganisms caused disease, he was involved in a study for the manufacturers of wine and beer. He was attempting to find out why wine and beer would at one time be good and at another time, not. During his studies he found that holding juices at a temperature of 145° F for 30 minutes would not harm the flavor but would inactivate undesirable microbes. The result was a consistently good product. Today, this process is called *pasteurization* in his honor.

Many scientists were attempting to link infectious disease with airborne microorganisms prior to and during the time Pasteur was experimenting with the germ theory of disease. Oliver Wendell Holmes, a Boston physician (1809-1894), theorized that puerperal (pu-er'-per-al) fever, or "childbed fever," was an infectious disease and the cause of many deaths among new mothers. He suggested that all persons attending deliveries wash their hands before treatment of each patient. His colleagues, not having read about what was going on in Europe, scoffed at him. This angered Holmes and he wrote a very indignant paper, "The Contagiousness of Puerperal Fever," which was largely ignored until about 1847. It is now a landmark in the history of medicine and has contributed much to the introduction of aseptic techniques in obstetrics and surgery.

About the same time (1846), a Hungarian physician, Ignaz Phillipp Semmelweis (Sem'-el-vis) (1818-1865), angered by the high death rate of mothers in obstetric wards, was also exploring the use of antiseptics and the effect of washing hands with chlorinated lime between cases. Those who listened to Semmelweis and washed their hands before treatment of each patient found that the number of deaths in new mothers was greatly reduced; but there were still the doubters, and it wasn't until Lister's works (1865) became well known that the use of antiseptics during surgery became common. Semmelweis, an enemy of dirt, died of the very blood poisoning he fought so hard to prevent.

During these times death was frequent due to infection following surgery. Joseph Lister (1827-1912), an English surgeon, hearing about Pasteur's findings and impressed by the similarity between wound infections and certain putrefactive changes that Pasteur had proved were caused by microorganisms, set out to prove that wound infection was due to microorganisms. Few disinfectants were known at this time, and after trying many, Lister hit upon carbolic acid (phenol). He diluted the acid and soaked surgical dressings in the solution; wounds did not become infected but healed rapidly. This was the establishment of today's aseptic (bacteria-free) technique.

In the latter part of the same century, Robert Koch, a German physician (1843-1910), fascinated by bacteriology, observed that there were deaths of many animals, and at times also the death of farmers, from anthrax. He suspected a microorganism was the cause. So he first observed, then grew and isolated, the anthrax bacilli in pure culture, and then injected the microorganism into experimental mice, which subsequently developed symptoms of anthrax. His next step was to recover the bacilli from the spleen of the experimental animal and confirm the identity of the microorganism causing anthrax. The result of these experiments proved conclusively that certain bacteria produce specific diseases. This experiment resulted in the publishing of *Koch's Postulates* (1876), which are today used as the basis of experimental investigations of infectious diseases (see following list).

Koch's Postulates

1. A specific organism must be observed in every case of the disease.
2. The organism must be isolated in pure culture.
3. The organism must, when inoculated into a susceptible animal, cause the disease.
4. The organism must be recovered from the experimental animal and its identity confirmed.

NEW WORDS

Normal flora: Resident bacteria primarily in the oral cavity and in the intestinal tract. As long as the resistance of the host is maintained at a high level, the "normal flora" do no harm.

Phenol: A dilute of carbolic acid.

SELF—TEST

1. Define microbiology. _____

2. What is the resident microbial population of the human body called?

   _____

3. What was the name of the Dutch scientist who ground microscope lenses perfect enough to see tiny creatures moving in rainwater? _____

4. What was the theory of spontaneous generation? _____

5. Who was the first scientist that attempted to disprove the theory of spontaneous generation? The second? Were they successful? _____

   _____

6. Who finally disproved spontaneous generation and established the "Germ Theory of Disease"? What other discovery did this scientist make? _____

   _____

7. Who was the first American to suspect that unwashed hands contributed to childbed fever? _____

8. What European physician had already explored the use of antiseptics to cut down deaths among new mothers? _____

9. Who finally proved that aseptic technique was the only way to eliminate death due to wound infection? What was the disinfectant used? _____

   _____

10. What German physician isolated and proved that a specific bacterium causes a specific disease? What procedures did he publish? Name these procedures in correct order. _____

    _____

Microorganisms are everywhere: fortunately most are harmless, and many are actually needed. To study these minute plants and animals, scientists developed methods of growing (culturing) microorganisms in great numbers, staining them, and then studying their morphology, metabolism, motility (ability to move), and their pathogenicity (ability to cause disease). These studies employed all methods available, including the use of the microscope and experimental animals.

Today, scientists continue to experiment with research that is very controversial—such as the creation of new life forms through cutting and splicing molecules of DNA, the substance that carries all hereditary information.

Methods of Identification and Classification

Microscopes. The method most frequently used to study minute organisms is the microscope, which may be a simple, compound, or electron microscope. The *simple* microscope is not much different from a magnifying glass. The *compound* microscope, consisting of two lens, is more useful, although the organisms must be rather large to be viewed. The *electron* microscope, through tremendous magnification, has revealed minute structures never before seen.

Staining. There are some bacteria so small they must be stained with special dyes to be seen through a microscope. In general there are three different classes of stains: (1) simple, (2) differential, and (3) special; of these three, only the *Gram stain*, a differential stain, will be discussed.

Christian Gram (1884) quite by accident discovered and then introduced to the scientific world the Gram-stain method of bacterial identification. He stained a bacterial smear with crystal violet, treated it with a weak solution of iodine, and then washed it with alcohol. He noted that some of the bacteria retained the stain: these he called *Gram-positive*; those that did not, he called *Gram-negative*.

Culture. Growing or culturing bacteria on artificial food (media) is an important method of studying and identifying microorganisms. Many times the microscope alone does not reveal all the necessary data. One method of studying a culture is first to inoculate sterile medium in a petri dish (a circular glass or plastic dish about 3 inches in diameter and ½ inch high) with bacteria. The petri dish is then incubated 24 to 48 hours, and the colonies that result will give much additional information. Some chromogenic bacteria such as *Staphylococcus aureus* will produce a colony that is golden yellow. Other microorganisms will produce colors specific to the individual strain. Some bacteria retain the color, and some excrete color into the surrounding medium. Through observation of the above characteristics one can further classify the microorganisms being observed. Yet another form of bacteria

213

will produce *hemolysins*. These are bacteria that destroy red blood cells. When grown on media, these bacteria can be identified through observation of colonies on blood agar plates. The red blood cells have been lysed (destroyed), and there is a clear zone around the colonies of hemolytic bacteria. From these brief examples you can see the importance of this technique of identification of bacteria.

Tissue Culture. Animal inoculation and tissue cultures from animals are also important links in the chain of disease identification and control. Tissue culture is used as a medium for propagating viruses. Animal inoculation is used in experimental and diagnostic virology. It is the introduction of a disease agent into a healthy individual to produce a mild form of the disease. These methods are used to identify, isolate, and determine the virulence (ability to cause disease) of specific organisms. This method of study (animal inoculation) is also basic to the manufacture of antitoxin (a particular kind of antibody produced in the body in response to the presence of a specific toxin).

Types of Microorganisms

Microorganisms are very selective in their environment, and to some the amount of oxygen present is very important for growth or survival. Scientists have used this need for oxygen to further identify specific organisms, and essentially to place them into two classifications: (1) those that need oxygen (aerobes), and (2) those that do not (anaerobes).

Aerobes. Aerobic bacteria live and grow in the presence of free oxygen (the majority of streptococci fall into this group.

Facultative Aerobes. Facultative aerobes can live in the presence of oxygen, but they do not require it. The majority of the staphylococci are in this category, for they grow best in the presence of oxygen but can grow in its absence also.

Strict or Obligate Aerobes. Strict or obligate aerobes cannot live without oxygen. The diphtheria bacillus is one organism that must have free oxygen to produce toxin.

Anaerobes. Anaerobic bacteria grow best in the absence of oxygen. *Fusobacterium fusiform* is just one example. This organism is found in ulcerative gingivitis (trench mouth).

Facultative Anaerobes. Facultative anaerobes grow best in the absence of oxygen but do not require its absence.

Strict or Obligate Anaerobes. Strict or obligate anaerobes cannot live in the presence of oxygen. One example is *Clostridium tetani*. These bacilli are found in soil, especially in farm lands where manure is prevalent. The bacillus enters through a break in the skin, particularily a puncture wound, causing an acute infectious disease that will often lead to death. *Clostridium botulinum* is also a strict anaerobe. The bacillus will grow where air cannot penetrate, as in canned food. If the food is not properly processed, the *Cl. botulinum* will give off toxin that often proves fatal.

Spores. Only a few organisms, primarily the bacilli, have the ability to form a hard resistant mass within the bacterial cell. This mass, called a *spore*, appears to be nature's method of perpetuating the vegetative form by hibernation; for it is only during times that are unfavorable for growth that a spore will form within the vegetative bacterial cell. After the spore has completely formed, the rest of the vegetative cell will disintegrate, leaving only a very resistant body (spore), which has been known to survive all kinds of adverse conditions for many, many years. However, when the hibernating spore is placed in an environment that is favorable for growth, the cell wall will rupture and a new vegetative cell, exactly like the original cell, is born. With the birth of the new cell, the process of binary fission takes place and continues until unfavorable conditions for growth are again met; then the process of hibernation is repeated. Two of the spore-forming bacteria that might be of concern in the dental office are those that cause tetanus and gas gangrene. Not all bacilli that form spores are pathogenic; and there are pathogens that do not form spores that are also of great concern to those in dentistry. However, it must be remembered that those that do form spores are more difficult to destroy.

Special Characteristics

Capsule. The slimy, gelatinous coating surrounding many bacterial cells is called a *capsule*; it may be thick or thin; it may be present one time and not another. However, it has been observed that when a bacterial cell is encapsulated, it is more virulent, and that the capsule also appears to protect the bacterial cell against the body's natural defenses. It has also been noted that when an encapsulated pathogenic cell loses its capsule, it also loses its ability to cause disease. When searching for the causative factor of disease, one must consider the chemical composition of the capsule since it is always specific to one bacterial cell, which makes this observation just one more method of identifying a specific bacterium.

Motility. Motility is another characteristic of bacteria that helps, somewhat, in identification. It is not an absolute, however, as there may be too many variables. The organ, or organs, of movement for the majority of the bacilli and spirilla are called *flagella*[1]. These long, thin, hairlike attachments extend from the outside of the cell. There may be one, two, or many. The number

[1] Cocci are another type of bacteria, spherical in shape. They are seldom motile.

of flagella and degree of motility differ between cells. Most motile cells move rapidly. The environment also will somewhat affect the amount of movement.

SELF—TEST

1. Define motility. _____

_____

2. Define pathogenicity. _____

_____

3. What essentially are the three types of microscopes? _____

_____

4. What is the Gram stain? Who developed it? _____

_____

5. Briefly list the three basic steps in a Gram stain. _____

_____

6. What is the term given to bacteria that retain the Gram stain? _____

7. What is the term given to bacteria that lose the Gram stain? _____

8. Does the Gram stain indicate pathogenicity? _____

9. Name four methods used to study microorganisms. _____

_____

10. Do some bacteria produce specific colors that aid in identification? What are these bacteria called? _____

11. What are bacteria called that will leave a clear zone around a colony on a blood agar plate? _____

12. What are bacteria that live and grow in the presence of free oxygen called? _____

13. What are bacteria called that can live in the presence of oxygen but do not require it? What are bacteria called that cannot live with oxygen? ____

_____

14. Name the bacteria that grow best in the absence of oxygen; that grow best in the absence of oxygen but do not require its absence and those that cannot live in the presence of oxygen. _____

_____

15. Which group of bacteria primarily have the ability to form spores? _____

16. Is this a form of hibernation? _____

17. Can the cell become viable again when conditions are favorable for growth? _____

18. What is the slimy gelatinous coating surrounding many bacterial cells?

_____

19. What are the organs that enable bacteria and spirilla to move? _____

MORPHOLOGY AND CHARACTERISTICS OF MICROORGANISMS

Characteristic Shapes

Van Leeuwenhoek's well-ground lens was the beginning. With the improvement of both lens and microscope, man's knowledge of the size, shape, internal and external structures, processes of division, and other characteristics of bacteria increased. The lens van Leeuwenhoek ground was powerful enough to allow him to see "tiny creatures that were prettily a-moving." He made accurate drawings of what he saw and gave accurate descriptions of the three shapes he observed. The three different shapes that he saw we now recognize as (1) the round *cocci* (Greek for "berry"), (2) the rod-shaped *bacilli* (Greek for "rod"), and (3) the curved, wavy, or coiled bacteria known as *spirilla, vibrios,* and *spirochetes*. Descriptions of these three forms are given below.

Cocci [coccus, singular]. The *micrococcus* is a single bacterial cell that is *round* in shape. *Diplococci* (*diplo* meaning "two") is made up of two cocci that remain together after fission (dividing). *Streptococci* (*strepto* meaning "chain") are those cocci that cling together in long chains as they divide. *Staphylocci* (*staphlo* meaning "cluster") are those cocci that form clusters like grapes.

Bacilli [bacillus, singular]. The bacillus is rod-shaped, with the rod differing in shape and size from species to species. These rod-shaped bacilli are generally single and unattached.

Spirillaceae (spi-ril′-lā-se-e). The spirillaceae are *spiral-shaped* forms that come in three subtypes.

1. Spirilla [spirillum, singular]. Spirilla are rigid, unattached individual cells that will differ in length, with some short and tightly coiled and others long and with many twists and curves. The number, size, and rigidity will also vary.
2. Vibrios [vibrio, singular]. Vibrios are small and curved organisms. They look very much like commas.
3. Spirochetes [spirochete, singular]. The spirochetes are similar to the spirilli, with one exception: they are not rigid. They can bend and twist as they move.

Five Main Groups of Microorganisms

There are five main groups of microorganisms. Each group has different characteristics, including different modes of reproduction. There also are variations in modes of reproduction within a group. The five groups are: the bacteria, fungi, rickettsia, viruses, and animal parasites.

Bacteria. Bacteria are one-celled plants that do not contain chlorophyll. Therefore, they cannot generate energy and nourishment from the sun as do plants that contain chlorophyll. (This ability of some plants to generate energy from the sun is called *photosynthesis* (fō″-tō-sin′-the-sis).) Therefore, to obtain nourishment and energy needed for growth, bacteria must rely upon their ability to break down organic matter into simpler chemical substances. This self-synthesis of organic matter into simpler chemical substances is called *chemosynthesis* (ke″-mo-sin′-thē-sis). Organisms that obtain their energy in this manner are classified as *heterotrophic organisms*. This group contains all of the pathogenic organisms dangerous to man.
Organisms that are capable of building up inorganic substances into organic substances are known as autotrophic organisms. All green plants and some bacteria are autotrophs. They are capable of both photosynthesis and chemosynthesis.
A special characteristic of bacteria that promotes their growth and assures them a place on this planet, from here to eternity, is their ability to select associated species that permit them to accomplish harmful or beneficial results that they cannot accomplish alone. This ability of working together to create a greater effect is known as *synergism*. Another characteristic that assures bacteria immortality is *symbiosis*, which refers to two dissimilar organisms that exist together (1) for the mutual benefit of each other (*mutualism*); (2) for the benefit of one but not detrimental to the other (*commensalism*); or (3) for the benefit of one and inhibiting the growth of another (*antagonism*): these three characteristics are all representative of *symbosis*.
Bacteria, as already mentioned, occur in three characteristic forms: the cocci, the bacilli, and the spirillaceae. When surroundings are favorable for growth, bacterial reproduction (binary fission) takes place. The cell multiplies until it divides, forming two identical cells. This division occurs approximately every 20 minutes. A *colony* (group of like cells) may form in as little as 18 hours. Without nature's methods of slowing or halting growth, trillions of bacteria could be present in 24 hours—a sobering thought. Some of the infections caused by cocci, bacilli, or spirillaceae are syphilis, gonorrhea, erysipelas, impetigo, cellulitis, tetanus, gas gangrene, diphtheria, and tuberculosis.

Fungi. The fungi are parasitic organisms in the plant kingdom that, like the bacteria, do not contain chlorophyll; so they, too, cannot produce their own food. Therefore, they must maintain life by existing on other living organisms or on the dead remains of plants and animals. The fungi vary in size from mushrooms, which are quite large, to a single cell that is so small it can be seen only through a microscope. Fungi, like other microorganisms, may be either beneficial or harmful to man. One disease that occurs in the oral cavity that is a result of fungi is thrush (moniliasis), which is caused by the yeastlike organism *Candida albicans.* This disease appears as whitish spots, or areas, on the red, moist, and inflamed mucous membrane. These organisms are present in persons in small numbers as part of the normal human flora. Thrush may be associated with a prolonged administration of antibiotics, which causes a decrease in the numbers of bacteria that would ordinarily suppress the growth of *C. albicans.* It is believed by some that fungi might be transferred by contaminated fingers, instruments, clothing, dust, or other fomites.

The fungi are divided into two subgroups: the yeasts and the molds.

Yeasts. Although small, yeasts are many times larger than bacteria. For the most part they are beneficial to man: they provide leavening for bread, and they also provide alcoholic beverages through the conversion of fruit juices (sugars) into alcohol. They reproduce in two ways. (1) The asexual process is by *budding*, where a daughter cell will form on the outer surface of the parent cell and cling there to allow fluid from the parent cell to enter. This fluid is forced into the daughter cell until it reaches the size of the parent cell; separation then occurs and a new cell called an asexual spore has been formed. (2) All "true" yeasts are produced by a process called *sporulation*, a sexual process where fusing may take place just prior to or immediately after spore formation. It may be the fusing of two similar cells or of two different cells. The cells containing the spores are enclosed in a sac that may contain anywhere from one to eight spores. These spores have been formed by repeated division of the nucleus into spores that will retain part of the original cell nucleus, later to be released as budding cells.

Molds. Molds, like yeasts, are for the most part beneficial to man. They are used in the manufacture of antibiotics; one of the best-known antibiotics is penicillin. However, molds are also useful in the manufacture of certain food products, of which citric acid is an example. This chemical is used in various medicines, flavorings, food, ink, and many other things. The reproductive process of molds is somewhat more complicated than the reproduction of bacteria and yeasts. One method is the forming of colonies that are covered with mycelia (filamentous threads), some of which grow up into the air to form reproductive cells or spores. Molds also reproduce by fragmentation (the scattering into numerous and widely scattered fragments). Molds, at times, also reproduce by budding. There are many pathogenic fungi. Ringworm and thrush are the most important in the dental office.

Rickettsias. The rickettsias are larger than the largest virus but smaller than the smallest bacteria, with an internal structure that is similar to bacteria. They divide by binary fission, but they cannot reproduce in the absence of living cells. They are parasites, and they are transmitted by way of infected insects to man. Some of the diseases that may be transmitted by the bite of an infected insect are fevers such as typhus, Q fever, and Rocky Mountain spotted fever.

Viruses. Viruses are the smallest of living organisms. They only cause disease in living tissue. Many diseases of man, lower animals, insects, and plants are caused by viruses. Like rickettsias, viruses can reproduce only inside living cells. They do not divide, as does the bacterial cell, but enter and infect the host cell where production of new viruses is stimulated. The host cell then disintegrates, releasing a new generation of viruses, resulting in such disesases as smallpox, herpes, respiratory infections, mumps, measles, polio, and on and on. One viral disease that is becoming more and more prevalent is hepatitis. This disease is of great concern to dentistry, for the chance of transmitting this disease from dentist and the auxiliary personnel to patient and vice versa is extremely high. Unfortunately, man is the host for most of the viral diseases that may be spread by either direct or indirect contact. These diseases cannot be treated with antibiotics; therefore prevention is most important. Proper immunization and precise sterilizing techniques must be adhered to.

Animal Parasites. Animal parasites are small organisms called *protozoa*, and they must live within or upon another living organism called the *host*. A tapeworm such as the beef tapeworm larva may enter man when underdone beef is ingested, and then continue to live on in the intestinal tract. To prevent acquiring any larvae from the *helminth* (worm) group, all beef, pork, or fish must be well cooked. Other parasites in this group, such as hookworm, may enter the human through the skin of the feet of those who go barefoot. The *Entamoeba coli* is a parasite that is found in the intestines of man. It is not considered pathogenic, although it is sometimes found in the inflamed tissues of periodontitis. These parasites reproduce by dividing lengthwise to form two new cells (binary fission).

SELF—TEST

1. Name the three different shapes of bacteria. _____

2. Name the five different groups of microorganisms. _____
   _____

3. Are bacteria plants or animals? _____

4. What is meant by the following? Be brief.
   (a) Photosynthesis. _____
   (b) Chemosynthesis. _____
   (c) Heterotrophic. _____
   (d) Autotrophic. _____

5. Into what group do the pathogenic organisms fall? _____

6. What term is used when bacteria work together to reach a certain goal?

_____

7. What term is used when bacteria exist together for their mutual benefit?

_____

8. What term is used when bacteria exist together to benefit one but not be detremental to the other? _____

9. What term is used when bacteria exist together and one is benefited but the growth of the other is inhibited? _____

10. What do all these terms refer to? _____

11. Are fungi parasitic or saphrophytic organisms? _____

12. What disease in the oral cavity is caused by a yeastlike organism? _____

13. How do yeasts reproduce? Molds? _____

14. How do bacteria reproduce? _____

15. Are rickettsias parasites? _____

16. Can viruses be cultivated outside of living tissue? _____

17. What disease caused by a virus is of great concern to dentistry? _____

18. Will antibiotics destroy viruses? _____

19. What are animal parasites, and how do they reproduce? _____

THE CAUSE AND PREVENTION OF DISEASE

We are surrounded by great numbers of microorganisms (about 1,600 have been identified); fortunately only a few (about 70) are *pathogenic* (able to cause disease), and only a dozen or so of these are dangerous. The majority of the microorganisms in our world are *saprophytes* (sap'-ro-fītes), which live on dead or decaying matter outside the human body and generally do not cause disease. In fact, many of these organisms are of great value to man. However, there are a few saprophytes that are pathogenic. One example is the saprophytic bacillus *Clostridium tetani* that causes tetanus (lockjaw) by entering the body through a puncture wound, invading the anaerobic environment and releasing its toxin into the surrounding damaged tissue.

Bacteria that produce toxin (poison) do so in two different ways. Some contain the toxin within the cell and are able to release the toxin only after the cell has been destroyed: these are *endotoxins*. Other bacteria release toxin through the cell wall into the surrounding environment: these are *exotoxins*. The *Clostridium tetani* and the *Clostridium botulinum* are examples of bacteria that produce exotoxins. The toxin of the *Clostridium botulinum* bacillus is so virulent that it can turn even a taste of canned food that has been poorly processed into a lethal weapon capable of killing. Endotoxin produced by the *Salmonella typhosa* bacilli (typhoid fever) appears to be released from the cell by the body's own defense system. An example: When an endotoxin-producing microorganism enters the proper host through the proper port of entry, the body's defenses are activated, and the invader (antigen) is enveloped and destroyed, at which time a specific toxin is released to cause a specific disease—in this case, typhoid fever. To cause the disease, however, the pathogenic organisms must enter the host in sufficient numbers to introduce toxin in quantities too great for the body's defense system to destroy.

Transmission of Disease

Each species of microorganism has a specific "port of entry" into the body. Some enter only through the skin; some through the respiratory tract or the digestive tract; and at least one (venereal disease), through the genito-urinary system. Syphilis, a venereal disease, cannot only be transferred in this manner by direct bodily contact, but it can also pass the placental barrier to infect the newborn child. Dentistry is concerned with those diseases that can either be introduced into or transmitted from the oral cavity, nose, skin, or inanimate objects (fomites), either by direct or indirect contact, during dental treatment. All dental personnel must pay strict attention to cleanliness and sterilizing techniques to prevent this cross-contamination.

Nature provided the human body with a strong defense system, but like all systems, there are times when a weakness within the system occurs. This is when pathogenic microbes strike. Generally pathogens have a specific method of transmitting disease. Some of them transmit disease by *direct contact*, which at times means *actual body contact* as in the case of venereal diseases; but it can also mean disease transmitted by *droplet infection* when the infected person coughs or sneezes. These airborne particles, coming from the mouth or nose, may float in the air for a long time; or they may lodge in the dust on the floor, only to be airborne when the dust is stirred, to again cause disease. *Blood transfusions* are also a form of transmission by direct contact.

Transmission of disease by *indirect contact* occurs when disease has been transferred by contaminated hands and inanimate objects, such as instruments, cups, etc. Yet another way that disease may be transmitted is through the bite of an *infected insect* that carries the organism within its body. Then of course there are the insects that carry pathogenic organisms on their feet or other parts of their bodies. Flies are big offenders. It has been estimated that flies carry at least 20 known diseases, of which typhoid fever is one. And last but not least, are the *human carriers*, the persons who harbor pathogens in their bodies but show no signs of illness. These may be persons convalescing from a disease or those who harbor the organism for a long time after recovery. Some of the diseases spread in this fashion are diphtheria, typhoid fever, dysentery, streptococci infections, pneumonia, and hepatitis. Unfortunately, diseases are difficult to eradicate entirely, because carriers of disease are difficult to identify, and thus epidemic diseases are kept alive. Animals also spread disease to man; in fact, there are 150 known pathogenic diseases that may be spread in this manner.

The Body's Natural Defense System

Nature was foresighted when planning the survival of the human race and placed at every "port of entry" to the inner body certain defenses to prevent elimination of the species. It is only when the body and these defenses have been weakened through poor care that pathogens are able to enter, release their toxin, and in some cases destroy the host.

Certain persons are natually resistant to particular pathogens because of their race, and others appear to be individually resistant or immune to specific pathogens; but all persons, regardless of race or degree of natural immunity, have body defenses to protect them. The outer layer of *skin* (epidermis) and the *mucous membrane* that lines the body's external cavities are the body's first line of defense. Very few microorganisms are able to break through these barriers when they are intact. Organisms that attempt to enter the eyes are many times not able to do so because of the eyelid's protection. If they do succeed in entering, tears will wash most of them away and down the nose. Those few that might escape the flood of tears are eliminated by a bactericidal substance called *lysozyme*. Pathogens that enter the nose or oral cavity are entrapped by the sticky mucous membrane and the cilia that line the nose, trachea, and bronchi. The intruders are then destroyed or ejected. The saliva in the oral cavity also has a bactericidal effect. If pathogens are swallowed, they are trapped by the mucous membrane that lines the esophagus; and if they reach the stomach by chance, the acidity of the gastric juices will destroy most of them. When pathogens do manage to overcome the body's first lines of defense, they are met by the *leucocytes* (white blood cells). These cells have the ability to go wherever they are needed. They are scavenger cells in the blood that with the help of certain *antibodies* engulf and ingest foreign particles. This action is called *phagocytosis*. However, with all of these elaborate defenses, pathogens do enter and do produce disease that is sometimes fatal. So man has long sought further protection from the pathogens.

Edward Jenner (1796), an English physician, noted that milkmaids who contracted cowpox, also called *vaccinia*, were immune to smallpox. Jenner reasoned that perhaps other persons could be made immune to the dread small pox if a small amount of the substance from a cowpox pustule on the hand of a milkmaid was applied to their arms. Without ever having seen the causative organism, Jenner set about his experiment. He transferred some of the material from a cowpox pustule, on the hand of a milkmaid, to the arm of a small boy. Six weeks later the boy was inoculated with small pox and failed to develop the disease. This was the first vaccination. Jenner then vaccinated 23 persons; and when none of them contracted the disease, he reported his discovery. Today smallpox has been almost eradicated from the world. However, on March 22, 1977, about 500 miles from Manila in the Philippine Islands, it was reported that at least 18 persons had died of smallpox. This proves that vaccination programs must be maintained for total security.

Several years after Jenner's discovery, Pasteur was attempting to find the cause of chicken cholera. Quite by accident, he not only discovered the cause of the disease, but also discovered nature's methods of prevention. He found that the bacteria that had lost their ability to cause disease could still stimulate the host to produce antibodies that would give protection against subsequent exposure to the same virulent organism. This discovery has led to a better understanding of the body's natural defense system.

Methods By Which Immunity Is Acquired

Immunization has been known for about 200 years; it is one method of preventing disease. Many scientists, beginning with Jenner, Pasteur, Koch, and Roux (Rōōz), discovered various methods of protecting humans against specific diseases. One step toward eradicating the dread disease diphtheria was the discovery, by Emile Roux, French bacteriologist (1853-1933), and Alexandre Yersin, French bacteriologist (1863-1943), in 1888, that diptheria produced toxin. Later, in 1913, the German bacteriologist von Behring produced toxin-antitoxin from the diphtheria toxin, and a permanent active immunity against diphtheria was obtained in humans. Today the Schick test, a skin test for determining susceptibility to diphtheria is used first; and then if the person is susceptible, he is immunized with a vaccine.

Methods of prevention have progressed rapidly since those early days, and the spread of many deadly diseases is now controlled. As long as humans are constantly alert and are aware that active immunity must be maintained, all is well. However, complacency could lead to new epidemics of dread diseases from the past.

There are four general methods by which immunity is acquired, as listed below.

1. *Natural:* Natural immunity is the immunity one is born with. It may be due to the natural heritage of the individual, species, or race. Other factors such as diet, temperature, or metabolism may also be involved.
2. *Acquired:* Acquired immunity, also called *induced immunity*, is that which results from antibodies not normally present in the blood but which are induced either by placental transfer, by an attack of the disease, or by vaccination.
3. *Active:* Active immunity is produced by natural or artificial means. It may be produced by an attack of the specific disease or by injection of vaccines or toxoids.
4. *Passive:* Passive immunity is a short-term immunization that is produced by the introduction into the body's system of serum (antiserum) or antitoxin that already contains antibodies. And, because the body's own cells play no part in producing the antibodies, the person immunized is protected only as long as the antibodies remain in his blood, usually from four to six weeks.

The term *inoculation* is used, at times, to describe the process of rendering a subject immune to a specific disease. Inoculation is the act of introducing microorganisms, infective materials, serum, or other substances into tissues of living plants and animals. Another term that is often used is *vaccination*. This term is derived from the word *vaccinia*, or *vaccine*, the substance taken from cowpox pustules and first used by Jenner to prevent smallpox. Today the term *vaccination* means injection for the purpose of immunity.

NEW WORDS

Antibody: A protein that is produced in the body in response to invasion by a foreign agent (antigen) and that reacts specifically with it.

Antigen: Any substance not normally in the body that when introduced, stimulates production of antibodies that react specifically with it.

Inoculation (i-nok'-u-la'-shun): Introduction of pathogenic microorganisms into the body to stimulate production of antibodies and immunity.

Vaccination (vak'-si-na'-shun): Inoculation with weakened or dead microorganisms to develop immunity to a specific disease.

Vaccine: A suspension of attenuated or killed microorganisms (viruses, bacteria or rickettsiae), administered for prevention or treatment of infectious diseases.

Attenuation (ah-ten-u-a'-shun): The act of thinning or weakening; the alteration of the virulence of a pathogenic microorganism by passage through another host species.

SELF—TEST

1. Briefly define: pathogen, saprophyte, endotoxin, exotoxin. _____

_____

_____

_____

2. What route must microorganisms follow to cause disease? _____

_____

3. Name four routes that microorganisms can take in order to cause disease in the body of a human. _____

_____

4. Define *direct* and *indirect contact* in the transmission of disease. _____

_____

5. Name four methods by which the body's defense systems attempt to protect the host from destruction. _____

_____

6. Who was the first to use a substance from cowpox to prevent a disease, and how did he perform his experiment? What was the disease? _____

_____

7. Pasteur found that the host could produce a reaction which gave protection against future exposure to the same virulent organism. Name the reaction. _____

8. Name and briefly define four methods by which immunity is acquired.

_____

_____

_____

9. Define *immunization*. _____

10. What is the Schick test? _____

DESTRUCTION OF MICROORGANISMS

The dental office must not be a source of infection to patients or personnel. The oral cavity contains a microbial colony capable of transmitting some of the most dread diseases. Therefore, all personnel in the treatment area must be well versed in aseptic techniques. Until recently it was virtually impossible to sterilize the handpieces that hold the rotary instruments used in most dental procedures. However, some manufacturers are now offering handpieces that can be autoclaved (apparatus for using steam under pressure for sterilization). Many manufacturers are also offering disposable items that formerly were nondisposable and were frequently the source of infection. Therefore, it is continually becoming easier to maintain aseptic procedures during dental treatment.

The primary objective of dental personnel must be to sterilize all things used in patient treatment and then store everything in such a way that nothing will become contaminated. Sterilization can be accomplished in two ways. First, microorganisms can be destroyed by *physical means*; and second, they may be destroyed by *chemical means*. Some types of sterilization within these two methods only inhibit growth of the cell, while some types actually destroy it. Prior to selecting the method of sterilizing, personnel must recognize which method will be the most effective one. Therefore, they must be knowledgeable of certain terms, as listed below.

Asepsis: Asepsis means the absence of all pathogens.
Sterilization: Sterilization is the process of destroying *all* forms of life.

Disinfection: Disinfection means death of disease-producing organisms and the destruction of their products.

Disinfectant: A disinfectant is usually a chemical that will kill growing forms but will not kill spore-forming bacteria. It is usually used on inanimate objects as it is too strong to be applied, full strength, to body tissues. Examples of disinfectants would be iodine and phenol.

Antiseptic: An antiseptic is truly a diluted disinfectant. It will prevent the growth of microorganisms by inhibition.

Sanitize: To sanitize means to reduce the number of bacteria to a safe level and free the item from pathogens.

Bacteriostatic: Bacteriostatic means capable of preventing the growth and activity of bacteria. Bacteriostatic agents do not kill spores but are somewhat germicidal for some microorganisms.

Bacteriocidal: Bacteriocidal signifies that some bacteria, but not spore forms, are destroyed.

When Is a Microorganism Dead?

Each situation must be evaluated because it is not possible to sterilize all things using one procedure. In the use of a chemical agent, timing, strength, and age of the solution are important. In the use of heat, steam, chemical vapor, or gas, the time, temperature, and pressure are important. The kinds of organisms present, the amount of contamination, and the item being sterilized must also be considered. All these factors play a part in accomplishing the objective: the death of all microorganisms that might otherwise cause infection.

Hands cannot be sterilized, but the use of surgical soap containing hexachlorophene is useful, along with a *thorough mechanical scrub* with a brush. Scrubbing with soap and water is the *mechanical removal of microorganisms* and proteins such as blood and saliva from hand instruments, cups, rotary instruments, etc. If mechanical removal is performed thoroughly, as much as 90% of all contaminents can be removed. A toothbrush is ideal for cleaning small areas that are hard to get at. Before sterilization, or disinfection, one must remove all soap by rinsing; and to prevent dilution, one must remove the water by drying. If an ultrasonic cleaner is available, this will eliminate the necessity to scrub with soap and water, but the instruments must be rinsed free of all ultrasonic solution, dried, and then sterilized.

In addition to disinfection of instruments and hands, the disinfection of the mucous membrane, before injection, will help to eliminate the carrying of any oral microorganisms into the underlying tissues and possibly causing infection. Merthiolate (an organic mercury preparation) is sometimes used to disinfect the mucous membrane at the site of an intra-oral injection.

Methods of Sterilization

Sunlight. Sunlight is nature's method of sterilization. Many microorganisms are destroyed by ultraviolet light emitted by the sun. Some organisms will be destroyed very quickly and others only after many hours. Many hospitals have installed ultraviolet light in the operating rooms as a means of destroying airborne organisms.

Alcohol. Alcohol is widely used as a disinfectant in 70% solution. Isopropyl alcohol is thought to be superior to ethyl alcohol as it can be used full strength; it is less expensive and its sale is not subject to restrictions.

Chemical Agents. There are many so-called cold-sterilizing agents available; however, most are not effective against spores, some bacilli, and some viruses. Chemical agents that are effective as disinfectants are those that contain chlorine (bleaching solution); disinfectants containing phenol; or a solution that contains formalin, alcohol, and hexachlorophene, which can kill all bacteria, spores, tubercle bacilli, and viruses, providing that time, age, and strength of the solution are constant. All chemical substances are rated according to their bactericidal activity in relation to phenol. This is called the *phenol coefficient*.

The disinfection of instruments and surfaces in and around the treatment area is a very real problem. Many pathogenic organisms are found in the dental environment. These organisms can cause serious infections, some of which are tuberculosis, syphilis, tetanus, and—one that is becoming almost epidemic—hepatitis. This last one, hepatitis, is of great concern to dentistry. All dental personnel should protect themselves with masks and gloves when treating a patient with a history of serum hepatitis. All items used around a hepatitis patient should be disposable. Those that are not disposable should be autoclaved. Instruments or items that cannot be either disposed of or autoclaved should be soaked in a solution of 10% hypochlorite and 2% glutaraldehyde, a solution that is commercially known as Cidex. Spores can be destroyed by this solution in 3 to 5 hours. Chemical solutions such as Zepherine and benzyl are frequently used in dental offices. If used, they are most effective as disinfectants when alcohol is added to the solution. All these solutions must be changed frequently; and instruments placed in them must be clean, rinsed of soap, and dried. All instruments must be fully immersed for a minimum of 30 minutes, rinsed and dried, and stored in an area free from contamination. These solutions should not be used for sterilizing instruments such as scalers, scalpels, forceps, etc., that might possibly come in contact with blood.

Boiling Water. Boiling water is generally not used as a sterilizing procedure, although it will kill all microorganisms except spores and hepatitis viruses, in 10 minutes. To kill hepatitis viruses, articles must be boiled not less than 30 minutes, and more time is required to kill spores. Therefore, boiling water should be considered as a means of disinfecting rather than as a means of sterilizing items.

One disadvantage of this method of disinfection is that is will rust instruments unless a rust preventative is added. It will also dull instruments. Another disadvantage is the building up of deposits. Although the boiling-water sterilizer is emptied and dried each day, deposits will form inside, and then must routinely be removed. Before placing any instruments into the boiling water, add one cup of white vinegar and boil for 10 minutes; empty the boiling water bath, and all deposits will be easily removed.

Such items as needles and syringes, or any item that might enter the bloodstream, should not be placed in the boiling water; they should be sterilized in an autoclave.

To make this method more bactericidal it is possible to add to the boiling water a phenolic disinfectant.

All items, of course, must be cleaned before completely immersing them in the boiling water, and the water must be kept at a rolling boil during the disinfecting period.

Autoclaving. The autoclave (aw'-to-klāv) is self-locking equipment for sterilizing material by steam under pressure. The autoclave allows steam to flow around each article placed in the chamber. The *moist heat* will penetrate cloth or paper used to package articles being sterilized. Autoclaving is one of the most effective methods for the destruction of all types of micro-organisms. Temperatures of 250° F (121° C) to 270° F (126° C) at 15 to 20 lb pressure for 15 to 45 minutes will kill all organisms and spores, depending on what is being sterilized, the size of the load, and how it is wrapped.

The manufactures' directions for operating and care of each type of autoclave must be followed to ensure complete sterilization of all materials and to protect this expensive piece of equipment from damage.

Not all materials and instruments can be autoclaved. Two materials—fats and oils—or instruments that might rust or be dulled should not be auto-claved.

Dry Heat. Dry heat or hot-air sterilization in an oven (baking) is much slower than the moist heat of autoclaving. The dry-heat method is most often used to sterilize items that cannot be sterilized in any other manner. Items such as glassware, metal, petrolatum oils, and cutting instruments are some of the things that can be sterilized by this method.

All items should be packed loosely, with space between each package. The temperature must be uniform, with anywhere from 302° F (150° C) to 320° F (160° C) being most frequently used. This temperature is then held from 1 to 3 hours, depending on what is being sterilized and the size of the load. Care must be taken that higher temperature is not used when sterilizing some instruments as this could be the cause of solder melting and ruining the instruments. Aluminum foil is very good to use as a wrap since it conducts heat well and will not burn, as will cotton wraps. It is advisable to load an oven when it is cool; then allow the load to cool in the oven before removing it.

Unsaturated Chemical Vapor. The system of unsaturated chemical vapor depends on heat, water, and chemicals working together to form an unsaturated vapor that will not rust, corrode, or dull instruments, as does the saturated steam method (autoclave). This is a very effective method of sterilizing most items. Ideally, all items should be processed in a special-type paper sterilizing bag. However, they can be placed on a towel and either covered or not covered. Care must be taken not to load so many items at one time that the vapor cannot reach all parts of each item. All sterilized items must then be stored so that there is no chance of recontamination. If covered metal trays are to be sterilized, the cover must be removed. As with all methods of sterilizing, items must be dry and free of debris before sterilization.

The Harvey Chemclave is one of the best-known chemical vapor sterilizers. It is suitable for sterilizing most items used in the dental office. However, new pieces of equipment are constantly being placed on the market, and although the operation of each will be similar, the manufacturers' directions should be followed carefully.

Checking Performance. When sterilizing by dry heat, moist heat, or chemical vapor, one should use indicator strips to be certain that all items have been sterilized. There are special types of indicator strips for all types of sterilizing equipment. However, these should not be considered 100% foolproof. It has been suggested that every few months a spore strip be placed in the densest part of a load; then sent to a laboratory to determine whether all microorganisms are being destroyed. However, because all offices possibly cannot take advantage of this laboratory check, it is most important that the checks that are available be used.

Molten Metal and Glass Beads. Molten metal and glass beads are methods of sterilizing that are most often used in conjunction with endodontic treatment. They, like other methods, have both good and bad features. Molten metal can cause steel instruments to either lose or alter their temper, and paper points to become brittle; but the advantage is that it takes only 10 seconds to sterilize a file or reamer. There is a necessary precaution, however, and that is, all metal clinging to instruments must be removed by tapping against the container, as any metal clinging to the instrument could be carried into the pulp canal.

The glass bead sterilizer is filled with minute glass beads, or table salt. Instruments are inserted into a preheated container of glass beads. This method appears to be more popular than that of molten metal, the reasons being that the temperature is more easily controlled, and there isn't the danger of carrying foreign material into the canal. However, it does take a bit longer to sterilize the instruments, approximately 15 to 20 seconds for paper (absorbent points) and only 10 seconds more for cotton pellets.

General Office Procedures

More than at any time in the past, personnel in dental offices are becoming aware of the need to evaluate a patient's general physical condition. In many dental offices it is now routine to take a health history, check blood pressure, and do a complete examination of the head, neck, and oral cavity. Taking a patient's temperature is part of this work-up, and the oral thermometer must be sterilized. One method is to wipe the thermometer clean with a gauze square saturated with equal parts of a liquid surgical soap and 95% ethyl alcohol, to rinse well, and then immerse in a solution of 70% isopropyl alcohol for at least 10 minutes. To increase the effectiveness, 0.5% to 1% iodine might be added to the solution. Prior to use, the thermometer must be rinsed. If not used immediately, it must be rinsed, dried, and then stored in a sterile container.

Another item in the dental office that is frequently overlooked is the transfer forcep. This item can become a source of infection. It should be autoclaved daily, and should it become contaminated during treatment, it must be resterilized.

Everything that is handled during treatment is contaminated with saliva, which if not removed will dry, and the microorganisms present in some cases will remain active for long periods. Therefore, between patients, *all* surfaces should be wiped with cloths saturated in phenolic solution.

Many microorganisms that are capable of causing disease will remain in the dust in a treatment room and then become capable of causing disease when, in sufficient numbers, they enter the proper host through the proper port of entry. These are airborne microorganisms. Therefore, all items that have been sterilized must be covered to prevent contamination.

Converting Fahrenheit to Centigrade (Celsius)

Some of the equipment might possibly still be using Fahrenheit and some centigrade (Celsius); therefore, a brief discussion of conversion methods is presented.

To change Fahrneheit to centigrade, using 320°, do the following:

Method 1.

$$320° \text{ F} + 40 = 360 \times \frac{5}{9} = 1800 - 9 = 200 \text{ C} - 40 = 160° \text{ C}$$

$$\frac{\begin{array}{r} 320 \\ +40 \end{array}}{360} \qquad \frac{360}{1} \times \frac{5}{9} = \frac{1800}{9} = \frac{\begin{array}{r} 200 \text{ C} \\ -40 \end{array}}{160 \text{ C}}$$

To change centigrade to Fahrenheit, using $160°$ C, do the following:

$$160° \text{ C} + 40 = 200 \times \frac{9}{5} = 1800 - 5 = 360° \text{ F} - 40 = 320° \text{ F}$$

Method 2.

$$320° \text{ F} - 32 = 288 \times \frac{5}{9} = 1440 - 9 = 160° \text{ C}$$

$$\begin{array}{r} 320 \\ -32 \\ \hline 288 \end{array} \qquad \frac{288}{1} \times \frac{5}{9} = \frac{1440}{9} = 160° \text{ C}$$

$$160 \times \frac{9}{5} = 1440 - 5 = 288 + 32 = 320° \text{ F}$$

SELF—TEST

1. Can all handpieces be autoclaved? _____

2. Although cost might be a factor, is it still best to use disposable items? Why? _____

_____

3. Name two ways articles can be sterilized. _____

4. Define the following: asepsis, sterilization, disinfection, disinfectant, antiseptic, sanitize, bacteriostatic, bactericidal. _____

_____

_____

_____

_____

_____

_____

_____

5. Can all things be sterilized by one method? _____

6. There are three things that are important considerations when using a chemical agent to sterilize or disinfect. Name them. _____

_____

7. What is one method used to sanitize the hands? _____

8. What mechanical method is used to remove organisms before sterilization? Why is it important? _____

9. What other care must be given to all items before sterilization? _____

10. Name the disease of most concern to dentistry. How should personnel protect themselves from this disease? _____

11. What is Cidex? _____

12. To kill spores items should be immersed in this solution for how many hours? _____

13. Why is boiling water not considered as a means of sterilization, but only as a means of disinfection? _____

14. Should needles and syringes and surgical instruments be sterilized by: autoclave, chemical disinfectant, or boiling water? Circle one.

15. What is the temperature and pressure most often used in autoclaving? _____

16. Is it the moist heat or the pressure that does the sterilizing? _____

17. Will items, size of pack, and the organisms present regulate the time factor in autoclaving? _____

18. What are two disadvantages of sterilization by dry heat? _____

19. Is the chemical vapor method satisfactory? If so, why? And if not, why not? _____

20. Should all methods of sterilization have a check control to be certain sterilization is complete? _____

21. When is molten metal and/or a glass bead sterilizer used most often? _____

22. How is an oral thermometer sterilized? _____

23. Should the transfer forceps ever be autoclaved? _____

24. Is dust a factor in causing infection? _____

25. Convert 320° F to Celsius. _____

26. Convert 160° C to Fahrenheit. _____

Bibliography

American Institute of Biological Sciences, Biological Sciences Curriculum Study; *Biological Science, Molecules to Man*. Boston: Houghton Mifflin Company, 1963.

Broomell, I. Norman, and Philipp Fischelis, *Anatomy and Histology of the Mouth and Teeth*, 5th ed. Philadelphia: P. Blakiston's Son & Co., 1917.

Cook-Waite Laboratories, *Manual of Local Anesthesia in General Dentistry*. New York, 1972.

Frobisher, Martin, Lucille Sommermeyer, and Robert Fuerst, *Microbiology in Health and Disease*. Philadelphia: W. B. Saunders Company, 1969.

Gray's Anatomy of the Human Body, Charles M. Goss, ed., 29th ed. Philadelphia: Lea & Febiger, 1973.

Guyton, Arthur C., *Function of the Human Body*, 2nd ed. Philadelphia: W. B. Saunders Company, 1965.

Kimber, Diana, and Carolyn Grey, *Textbook of Anatomy and Physiology*. 7th ed. New York: The Macmillan Company, 1927.

Miller, B. F., and Claire B. Keane, *Encyclopedia and Dictionary of Medicine and Nursing*. Philadelphia: W. B. Saunders Company, 1972.

J. M. Ney Company, *Ney Bridge and Inlay Manual*. Hartford, Conn., 1954.

Orban's Oral Histology and Embryology, Harry Sicher, ed., 6th ed. St Louis, Mo.: The C. V. Mosby Co., 1966.

235

Pelszar, Michael J., Jr., and Roger D. Reid, *Microbiology*. New York: McGraw-Hill Book Company, 1958.

Schour, Issac, *Oral Histology and Embryology*, 6th ed. Philadelphia: Lea and Febiger, 1962.

Sicher, Harry, *Oral Anatomy*, 4th ed. St. Louis, Mo.: The C.V. Mosby Co., 1965.

Simpson, G. G., and W. S. Beck, *Life: An Introduction to Biology*, 2nd. ed. New York: Harcourt Brace Jovanovich, Inc., 1965.

Smith, Alice Lorraine, *Principles of Microbiology*, 5th ed. St. Louis, Mo.: The C. V. Mosby Co., 1965.

Webster's New Collegiate Dictionary, Springfield, Mass.: G. & C. Merriam Co., 1961.

Wheeler, Russell C., *A Textbook of Dental Anatomy and Physiology*, 4th ed. Philadelphia: W. B. Saunders Company, 1965.